The
Excruciating History
of
Dentistry

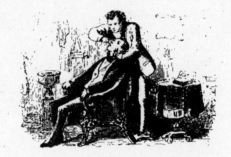

Also by James Wynbrandt

U2

Executive Retirement Management: A Manager's Guide to the Planning and Implementation of a Successful Retirement

The Encyclopedia of Genetic Disorders and Birth Defects

The Dan Quayle Diktionary

The
Excruciating History
of
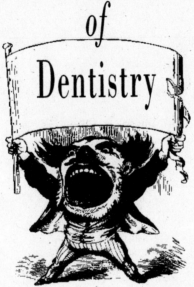
Dentistry

Toothsome Tales & Oral Oddities
from Babylon to Braces

♦

JAMES WYNBRANDT

St. Martin's Griffin ≈ New York

Artwork from the National Library of Medicine collection

THE EXCRUCIATING HISTORY OF DENTISTRY. Copyright © 1998 by
James Wynbrandt. All rights reserved. Printed in the United States
of America. No part of this book may be used or reproduced in any
manner whatsoever without written permission except in the case of
brief quotations embodied in critical articles or reviews. For information, address St. Martin's Press, 175 Fifth Avenue, New York,
N.Y. 10010.

Production Editor: David Stanford Burr
Design: Ellen R. Sasahara

www.stmartins.com

Library of Congress Cataloging-in-Publication Data

Wynbrandt, James.
    The excruciating history of dentistry / toothsome tales & oral
oddities from Babylon to braces / by James Wynbrandt.
        p.   cm.
    Includes bibliographical references and index.
    ISBN 0-312-18576-6 (hc)
    ISBN 0-312-26319-8 (pbk)
    1. Dentistry—History.   I. Title.
RK29.W86   1998
617.6'009—dc21   98-9794
                                                     CIP

D 10 9 8 7 6 5 4 3

Acknowledgments

The author wishes to thank the staffs and facilities of the New York University Dental Library; the library and Malloch Rare Book Room of the New York Academy of Medicine; the New York Public Library and its Rare Books and Manuscripts Division; the American Dental Association Library and the Dr. Samuel D. Harris National Museum of Dentistry; and to the many individuals who so freely shared their time and knowledge. Special thanks to Dr. John Hyson and Aletha Kowitz for their encouragement and assistance and to the members of the American Academy of the History of Dentistry for their inspiring dedication to the rediscovery and preservation of the profession's heritage. A deep debt of gratitude also to Charlie Spicer and Madeleine Morel, without whom this work would not have been possible.

Contents

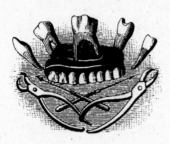

Introduction

THE DISTINCTIVE HIGH-SPEED GLISSANDO ASCENDING IN THE background. The peculiar odor of flavored antiseptic mingling with vaporized enamel. The clip from *The Marathon Man* that loops through the head and the tightening sphincter. Welcome to the dentist's office, an experience of sight, sound, smell, and sensation evoking a Proustian hell of remembrance.

As patients settle back into the contoured reclining chair—a direct descendant of the pioneering modern model now housed in the Smithsonian Institution—those who find the dental visit traumatic should consider how fortunate they actually are. Had their appointments been scheduled a little earlier—say, the first part of the twentieth century—they might have been blasted with dangerous levels of radiation or had a handful of perfectly good teeth pulled to promote general health. If, due to scheduling conflict, the visit had been moved up a couple of centuries, the patient might have been bled, blistered, or burned in the name of pain relief. Or the dentist might just as likely have administered a deadly dose of arsenic as recommended a simple urine rinse as a palliative. Or perhaps the patient might have found himself onstage before a lusty crowd, at the mercy of a tooth-drawer, the perfidious practitioner who is among the progenitors of this belatedly ennobled profession.

The legion of dental phobics and others whose whine rises in tandem with that of the drill would do well to stifle their terror and instead offer thanks to Apollonia, patron saint of toothaches sufferers. For today they face only fleeting discomfort rather than the disfiguring distress or slow agonizing death oft meted out by dental health-care providers of the past. The transition from yesterdays' ignorance, misapprehension, and superstition to the enlightened and nerve-deadened protocols of today has been a long, slow, and very painful process. Though study of this bloody and violent evolution may set one's teeth on edge, I can make a pledge regarding its reading that is typically dismissed out of hand when offered in a professional setting: This won't hurt a bit.

1

Demons, Worms, and Excess Fluids

Suspected Causes and Horrific Cures of the Ancient World's Dental Problems

THE ORIGINS OF THE ANCIENT HEALING ARTS KNOWN TODAY AS dentistry are obscure, a tale cloaked in equal parts mystery and misery. What is known is that throughout much of recorded time, dentistry has been advanced at the hands of inept practitioners, some with the best of intentions, others with the most venal motives. For dental patients, the clinical outcomes arising from these opposing approaches typically differed little. In either case, treatment for dental problems has historically been more bloody and barbarous than beneficial. If anything can blunt the sting of this painful fact, perhaps it is the recognition that in suffering dental distress and sundry oral afflictions, man is not alone.

Defective dentition has plagued living creatures for at least a quarter billion years—even before they had teeth. A fossil from a Devonian sea that submerged present-day Ohio some 250 million years ago records the oldest traumatic dental injury yet identified. The petrified remains of a fishlike creature twenty feet long bear the scar of an abrasion caused by its cuspidlike dental organs, as though the jaw had been unnaturally forced closed. We can only speculate what massive force could have caused such an injury, or how much it would cost to have it treated today.

Evidence of the more insidious destruction of decay goes back 100 million years. Fossils from the Permian period of the Paleozoic era show the unmistakable signs of bacterial invasion of periodontal tissue.

(A term that encompasses gums and bone that support the teeth, though in the case of fossils, the gums have long since receded.)

The earliest evidence of dental caries—tooth decay, in common parlance—dates to the same era, found in the tooth of a herbivorous dinosaur of the Cretaceous period. Fish of this period likewise endured a destructive process similar to caries.

We can deduce that periodontosis (bacterial destruction of the periodontal tissue) was rampant on land by the Miocene epoch of the Cenozoic era. The mandible of a three-toed horse of the period shows clear signs of destructive decay. Mighty mastadons also had dental problems, and so did camels, cave bears, and most other species of the time identified in fossil remains. Underscoring the severity of potential dental problems faced by ancient animals is the case of an impacted tooth in a saber-toothed tiger found in the La Brea tar pits in Los Angeles.

As the saber-toothed tiger sank into the tar, mired in pain, history awaited a creature capable of leaving a written record of its oral dilemmas and the woeful inadequacy of their treatment.

Of Caveman and Cavities

EARLY MAN WAS spared the misery of tooth decay; without refined sugar in his diet, caries were relatively rare. Nonetheless, toothaches and other dental maladies abounded. Most problems arose from excessive wearing of the teeth, caused by a combination of powerful jaw muscles and a coarse diet leavened with sand, dirt, and grit from grinding bowls. Extreme wear is seen in the dental remains of all prehistoric cultures. By the end of a caveperson's relatively short life, teeth were often so worn that the pulps were exposed. Bone loss indicative of severe gingivitis (gum disease) is also visible from remains.

As civilization arose, differences in diets of the wealthy and poor were evidenced in the state of their teeth. Typically, the richer the individual, the poorer their oral health, as decay made inroads in the human mouth. Thus, whether caused by wear or decay, the toothache has been mankind's primary dental affliction throughout history.

When teeth were good, however, they could be very, very good. They were thought to possess unusual healing powers and strong rejuvinative properties. Regarded as icons of health and life in cultures around the world, they served as emblems of vitality and even immortality. Teeth traditionally played an important role in the practice of magic, and were the most frequently and variously mutilated organs of the body. Tooth mutilation, from cosmetic filing to decorative inlays, has been practiced by peoples including Australian aborigines, Mongolians, Africans, the Papuans, Malayans, American Indians, Aztecs, and Mayans.

King Solomon, known for his wisdom, is said to have complimented Sheba on her set, exclaiming, "Thy teeth are like a flock of sheep that are even shorn, which come up from the washing." The poets and writers of Rome celebrated teeth as an asset to a woman's beauty and an orator's diction, though they also satirized the vain preoccupation with teeth.

We can assume dentistry was first practiced as were other forms of medicine, by a member of a priest class who used incantations, prayers, and amulets to affect cures. Who was the first to try his hand at this nascent healing art? The answer, as dental historian J. A. Taylor has written, "is shrouded in the mists of antiquity along with the history of the pyramids and other relics of early civilization." Indeed, little is known of dental history. Only recently has it become an object of interest. The first account of the subject written in English, *A History of Dentistry from the Most Ancient Time Until the End of the Eighteenth Century*, by Vincenzo Guerini, wasn't published until the twentieth century. Accurate records and documentation is rare, and accounts that exist are often suspect.

Ointments, salves, and other natural remedies no doubt played a role in these early ministrations, as they have throughout recorded history; along with reliance on spiritual leaders, dentistry also developed as an "empirical" medicine, whose practitioners sought knowledge from observing the natural world.

If a tooth required extraction, it was simply knocked out. A piece of hardwood, stone, or other rigid object was placed against the problem tooth, and struck with a rock or other malletlike instrument. Whoever first performed this procedure and wherever it was undertaken, it is certain to have aroused enmity. "Men did not like to have a useful and ornamental member of their bodies torn rudely from its socket," as Bernhard W. Weinberger pointed out in his seminal work on dentistry,

Orthodontics, an Historical Review of Its Origin and Evolution (1926), "and though they admitted its necessity since no means for a cure existed, still they could not feel grateful to the operator."

But what could bring such pain to so seemingly indestructible a body part? All cultures of the world attributed toothaches to one of three causes: Tooth demons, toothworms, or "humors," (fluids).

The demons were evil spirits, sent by the gods or cast by the spell of an enemy. The worms were believed to be small, maggotlike gnawing creatures. And the humors were the precious bodily fluids that if unbalanced, could create a host of health problems. The resulting therapies prescribed were typically brutal, often horrific, and not infrequently lethal. One must try to plug his ears to human suffering as the history of these treatments is recalled.

Tablets for Toothaches

"TAKE A TABLET and call me in the morning." That was the advice a Babylonian toothache sufferer might have been offered. Babylonians were battling toothaches as early as 5000 B.C. according to some accounts, and their therapies were recorded on cuneiform tablets.

Records recovered from the library of King Ashurbanipal in Nineveh and from Assur (Assyria), Nippur, and Uruk, reveal Babylonians blamed both demons and worms for toothaches. Initially the worm was thought to bore its way into teeth, a theory later giving way to a belief in its appearance by spontaneous generation, arising through putrefaction.

One story of the toothworm's genesis is found on a therapeutic tablet inscribed by the hand of Nabunadinirbu, son of Kudarnu. The "Legend of the Worm" provides directions for relief of Marduknadinachu—a toothache in contemporary dental nomenclature, by invoking Ea, god of the abyss and Anu, god of heaven, to smote the toothworm. This was accomplished by reciting an incantation that recounts the history of the creature:

As the God Anu created the sky, the sky created the earth, the earth created the rivers, the rivers created the canals, and the canals created the marsh. The marshes created the Worm, the Worm came crying before Shamash, the son, before

Ea, his tears streamed down. "What do you give me to eat?" I will give you dried figs or apricots. "For me! What is this? Dried figs or apricots? Let me insert myself in the inner of the tooth and give me his flesh for my dwelling. Out of the tooth I will suck his blood, and from the gum I will chew the marrow. So I have entrance to the tooth!" Because you have said this and have asked for, Worm, may God Ea strike you with the might of his hands. You shall pulverize henbane and knead it with gum mastic and place it in the upper part of the tooth, and three times you shall recite this incantation.

Toothache sufferers could also make direct appeals for relief through prayer:

O Shamash, because of my tooth which hurteth me, some ghost to whom I have not offered food nor poured forth water is angry. . . . To thee I pray that I may shut him in and cover him over, like a moth whose tooth hurteth him not, so shall (my) tooth, too, not hurt me."

Those whose pleas were answered joined a parade of formerly afflicted who hung clay tablets in temples, describing their ailments and what had been done to cure them. Priests compiled collections of the most important of these tablets. These compendiums may be regarded as among history's first medical textbooks.

One compilation of some forty tablets entitled, "When the conjurer goes to the house of the sick," offered a guide to diagnosis and prognosis of a panoply of ailments, organized by symptoms listed sequentially from head to toe. The teeth were used in the diagnosis of thirteen of the described medical problems. Though some of these tablets were damaged, a sample of what remains indicates how large a role teeth played in diagnostic protocols:

If his teeth are dark-colored, the disease will last a long time.
If one of his teeth aches and saliva flows, . . .
If his teeth are white, he will become well. . . .
If his teeth are dark-colored, the disease will last a long time.
If his teeth are crowded together, he will die.
If his teeth (fall out) his house will collapse.

If he grinds his teeth, the disease will last a long time. . . .
If he grinds his teeth and his hands and feet shake: Hand of
the moon god, he will die. . . .

One recovered tablet offered a cure for what we now know as brux-
ism, or grinding of the teeth:

> . . . take a human skull and spread a cloth of apple-colored
> wool across a chair. That skull you place on it. For three days,
> both morning and evening bring a sacrifice and recite seven
> times the conjuration into the skull. The skull should be kissed
> seven and seven times by the patient, before retiring: then he
> will become well.

Amulets of magic stones worn in leather pouches around the neck
were another popular remedy of the era. But more proactive steps were
being taken against the toothworm, as conjurers faced competition from
an arising professional class of physicians. These healers used empirically derived knowledge of plants and natural substances to fashion
cures.

By about 2250 B.C., physicians were smoking "worms" out of cavities using henbane seed kneaded into beeswax. The mixture was
heated on a piece of iron and the smoke directed to the cavity by a
funnel. Following this treatment, the cavity was filled with a cement of
powdered henbane seed and gum mastic.

Around the same time the first attempt at mixing law and medicine
appeared in the form of Hammurabi's Code. Written in the name of
the great ruler of Babylon, King-Physician and surgeon, and inscribed
on a stone pillar, the code marked the birth of medical jurisprudence.
Through its laws, we know that barbers of the time performed minor
surgical operations, including occasional tooth extractions. The code
established fees for physicians and punishments for unskilled and unsuccessful treatment. Penalties for malpractice seem stringent even by
today's standards. According to Hammurabi, "Should a patient lose his
life owing to an unsuccessful operation, the surgeon's two hands should
be struck off as punishment."

Several of the statutes involved the teeth, not surprising given the
value of the commodity. Paragraph 200 and 201 addressed punishments for knocking out teeth. The first states that "If a man knocks out

the tooth of a freeman, he shall have his own tooth knocked out." The second decreed, "If a man knocks out the tooth of a slave, he shall pay one half mine of silver."

The promulgation of Hammurabi's Code signaled a further turning away from superstition, conjurers, and priests in favor of physicians. When Herodotus, the peripatetic and somewhat unreliable historian of the ancient world visited Mesopotamia around 500 B.C., he reportedly found medicine being practiced by laypersons rather than priests.

Tablets from the seventh and eighth centuries B.C. reveal the Babylonians also developed humoral theories of medicine, that is, treatments aimed at restoring the balance of the body's humors: blood, yellow bile, black bile, and phlegm, as defined by the Greeks. These cures involved exorcisms of poisons through defecation, urination, sweating, blowing mucous from the nose, or in some cases the discharge of mother's milk.

Despite the attention to toothaches and laws regulating dental care, this was an orally uncivilized land; besides the rare extraction, there is no evidence that operative, restorative, or prosthetic dentistry was practiced in Babylon. Teeth weren't drilled, filled, or replaced, and bridges and dentures were unknown, all of which are viewed as hallmarks of civilization in the eyes of dental historians.

The Assyrians and Persians, like the Babylonians, were familiar with dental problems and prescribed similar methods of treatment. However, there is no convincing evidence they reached the level of civilization associated with the development of dental restorative arts, either.

The Bible evinces little interest or knowledge of dental medicine in its pages. The Talmud is likewise dentally disengaged, though it notes ancient Hebrews extracted teeth while advising against the practice. It also recommends holding a grain of salt in the mouth to relieve toothache. The tooth's power and glory were invoked in its well-known axiom, "an eye for an eye and a tooth for a tooth," and the less quoted adage, "If a man miste out one of his servant's teeth he shall let him go free."

The toothworm can also be found gnawing through its pages, recounted in the Hebraic Talmud from the second to sixth centuries A.D.

Land of Cataracts and Caries

TO THE LIST of plagues that afflicted ancient Egypt, add toothaches and periodontal disease. Extensive examinations of mummies have revealed that caries and abscesses began to appear regularly among aristocrats as early as 2500 B.C. The rise of a luxury class can be charted in the subsequent decline in dentition among Egypt's high society. Loss of teeth was common, with extensive, chronic, suppurative periodontitis—periodontal disease characterized by destruction of underlying bone—the most frequent cause.

These maladies did not arise for lack of care. Aristocrats had servants to attend the teeth as well as hair. Teethcleaning was so much a part of the morning ritual that the common parlance for "washing the mouth" became synonymous with the expression for breakfast. Physicians and specialists were respected and ubiquitous, and teeth were the object of serious attention. Of some 100 medical specialties, half a dozen were associated with dentistry, and dental specialists may have been practicing in Egypt as early as 3000 B.C.

The first hieroglyphic records of "one who deals with teeth" date to the time of King Djoser, in the Third Dynasty of the Old Kingdom, around 2600 B.C. Found inside a mastaba, or burial chamber, five wooden panels with portraits and titles proclaimed the entombed as Hesi-Re, "the greatest of those who deal with teeth [chief toother], and of the physicians." The hieroglyphic symbol for practitioners of the teeth was an eye and a horizontal elephant tusk. (Hieroglyphic evidence also exists for the trade of "tooth dealer," represented by a symbol similar to that of "one who deals with the hair.")

Besides being chief toother, Hesi-Re was guard of the diadem and director of royal records. Judging by the honors and titles bestowed on Hesi-Re and other Egyptian toothers, dentists were held in high regard. Khuwy, for example, was not only chief dentist, but also "Interpreter of the Secret Art of the Internal Organs" and "Guardian of the Anus."

Despite their esteem, the treatment options dentists offered were limited. They could alleviate some painful oral conditions and pathological lesions, but there is no record of them performing extractions, making prosthetic appliances, or replacing lost teeth. Thus, no convincing evidence exists that restorative dentistry was practiced on the mouths of the Nile.

Egyptians, like the Babylonians, first believed spirits were responsible for their afflictions. Amulets, magic spells, incantations, and prayers were part of the therapy protocol, as were a variety of purgatives, enemas, bleeding, diuretics, diaphoretics (to increase perspiration), and masticatories (chewed to increase salivation).

They wrote of oral disorders like "fire mouth," "blood eating" (thought to be a scurvy variant), "uxeda" and "bennet blisters in the teeth" (the latter two most likely abscesses or painful swelling). The remedies themselves could be dangerous, such as rinsing with a solution of colocynth. Made from the dried pulp of unripe fruit of the *Citrullus colocnythis*, this strong poison is a cathartic that modern texts say "has such drastic action that it should not be used." Egyptian dentists did, though they recommended watering down the potion with "evening dew."

Magic and superstition gave way to rational medical philosophy in the Middle Kingdom of 2000 B.C. But the age of reason was short-lived. As Egypt's power began to decline in about 1800 B.C., belief in gods and spirits as agents of disease reasserted itself, and the toothache demon again ruled the dental domain.

Prescriptive Papyrus

MUCH OF THEIR dental arts remained unknown to early Egyptologists, as mysterious and unfathomable as the Sphinx or the toothlike pyramids erupting from the nearby sands. Their secrets were finally revealed in about 1862, when German archeologist Georg Ebers was exploring the acropolis at Thebes, searching for antiquities to appropriate. There, between the crumbling thigh bones of a mummy, he discovered—surprise!—the Papyrus Ebers. Written about 1500 B.C., the early days of the New Kingdom (1552–1069 B.C.), the twenty-one meters of papyrus scroll catalog an accumulation of medical and dental knowledge extending back to perhaps 3500 B.C. Recorded in hieratic text, rather than the more cumbersome and conceptually limited hieroglyphics, it contains 700 remedies compiled by priests. A Rosetta stone of the healing arts, the Papyrus Ebers shows Egyptian familiarity with the pathology of the oral cavity: Inflammation, gingival abscesses, pulpitus—all are discussed.

The eleven dental remedies that Ebers describes consist primarily of plasters, mouthwashes, masticatories, and incantations. Loose teeth, rotting gums, and oral lesions receive prominent attention:

> The beginning remedies to fasten a tooth; powder of ammi/, yellow ochre/, honey/, are mixed together and the tooth is filled(?) therewith.
>
> Another to treat a tooth which gnaws against an opening in the flesh: cumin/, frankincense/, (untranslated)/, are pounded and applied to the tooth.
>
> Another to fasten a tooth: frankincense/, yellow ochre/, malachite/, are pounded and applied to the tooth.
>
> Another to expel eating on the gums and make the flesh grow: cow's milk/, fresh dates/, manna/, remains during the night in the dew, rinse the mouth for nine (days).

Frankincense and myrrh, in addition to making birthday gifts fit for a king, were highly valued for toothaches and other medicinal needs throughout the ancient world. Both are mentioned in the Papyrus Ebers. Frankincense, the gum resin from trees of the genus *Boswellia,* was also known as "thus" and "olibanum," derived from Hebrew "lebonah," which means milky, as was the tree's sap before it hardened into a resinous form.

Myrrh, the gum of the *Commiphora abyssinica* tree, took its name from the daughter of King Cinyrus of Cypress. Myrrh's story was told by Ovid, a torrid tale of unnatural passion. Lusting after her father, by deception Myrrh took her mother's place in his bed one night and became pregnant. When her father discovered her deception and its results, she was banished to the desert. Filled with remorse, she prayed not to be among the living or the dead. The gods answered her supplication and turned her into the tree that subsequently bore her name, its soothing sap said to be her tears of contrition.

Though myrrh's medicinal value is questionable, as late as 1951 it was listed in the tenth edition of the respected *Pharmacology and Dental Therapeutics,* recommended for use primarily for its aromatic properties.

The Papyrus Ebers also mentions the opium-yielding poppy in a long list of palliatives for toothaches, along with castor-oil plants (as an aspirant), calamine, caraway seeds, and arsenic. A recipe for an ointment used in extracting splinters is typical of the natural remedies of the era: "Cook the blood of womens, and mix it into oil. Then kill a mole, cook it and drain it in oil and follow by mixing the dung of an ass in milk. Apply the paste with the proper incantations."

Not all medications required such exotic ingredients. Another highly recommended general-purpose remedy was simple "water-in-which-the-phallus-has-been-washed."

The Edwin Smith Surgical Papyrus, found with the Ebers, but older by some seventy years according to some estimates, evinces more scorn for charms and magic formulas, reflecting the era of rationality in which it was written. Its toothache remedies include mudlike plaster packs for application to the affected area, concocted from ingredients as suited to an empty stomach as an oral cavity, such as dough, honey, fennel seeds, and onions. It also reveals knowledge of orthopedic dentistry, evidenced by the therapy for a dislocated mandible:

> *Thou shouldst put the thumbs*
> *Upon the ends of the Rami of the*
> *Mandible in the inside of his*
> *Mouth, and the two claws (two groups of four fingers)*
> *Under his chin and thou shouldst*
> *Cause them to fall back so that*
> *They come to rest in their places*
> *Though should bind it with y m r w (and)*
> *Honey every day until he recovers.*

Papyri discovered subsequently added to knowledge of dentistry in the time of the pharaohs and perhaps helped foster an image of the era presented by twentieth-century Hollywood. Anyone who's watched Boris Karloff lurch to life onscreen in a mummy movie, draped in a suit of linen strips, can appreciate the remedies suggested by the Papyrus Berlin for indeterminate dental pain:

> Smoke of twelve pieces of incense which one makes for one who suffers a toothache as a result of a whidu. Willow leaves and dry leaves of the sima plant are to be finely ground in myst-liquid and to be sprinkled with sweet beer. The Sufferer is to be fumigated with it and anointed.

Though history has lost the meaning of *whidu* and *myst-liquid,* the Egyptian fondness for fumigation is well documented. No orifice went unattended, as fumigants of one sort or another were commonly prescribed for a variety of oral, anal, and vaginal ailments.

When Herodotus visited Egypt he reported "Egypt is quite full of doctors; some attend to disorders of the eyes, others to those of the head, some take care of the teeth, others are conversant with all diseases of the bowels; while many attend to the cure of maladies which are less conspicuous." Though Herodotus's reputation renders the reliability of his account questionable, there is no doubt Egyptian dental specialists of the day would have been kept busy. Upper-class maladies of the mouth were trickling down to the masses. By the time of the Ptolemies (320–30 B.C.), caries were no longer rare among commoners. As Egyptians' oral health went into steep decline, so did their civilization.

Of Eastern Extraction

ANCIENT CHINESE WERE well acquainted with ya-tong—"toothache" to Anglophones—as well as caries. A dentally precocious civilization, they were more knowledgeable about oral afflictions than most contemporaneous cultures.

The origin of Chinese medicine is sometimes credited to Huang Ti, the Yellow Emperor. His book, *Neichung,* or *Canon of Medicine,* is said to have been written about 2700 B.C., though it was not published in a modern version until some time in the third century, B.C. But Emperor Shen Nung (ca. 3700 B.C.), also given credit for Oriental medicine's paternity, exhibited much more interest in teeth. His book *Pen Tsao* cataloged a cornucopia of medical treatments. (It has been revised and republished as recently as the mid-1950s.) For relief of toothache, he recommended mouthwashes, massage, herbal remedies, purgatives, and acupuncture.

Chinese medical texts identified nine distinct varieties of ya-tong, complemented by seven identifiable gum diseases. A hollow tooth, chung choo, was explained by the worm theory of cavitation, though humoral theories had their advocates, too. Records also reveal some ancient Chinese medical experts believed dental disease was caused by "excessive sexual intercourse." Perhaps this was an offshoot of the humoral theory, with depleted or unnaturally high levels of vital fluids being considered the causative factor.

Toothache treatments sometimes combined the rational and whimsical in inscrutable ways. Advised one, "Roast a bit of garlic and crush it between the teeth, mix with chopped horseradish seeds or saltpeter, make into a paste with human milk; form pills and introduce one into the nostril on the opposite side to where the pain is felt."

If the ache persisted, small arsenic pills placed near the tooth typically killed the pain, and with it probably the nerve, surrounding tissue, and possibly the patient as well.

Acupuncture was another recommended treatment, as it was for a variety of ills, making this among of the oldest forms of dental or oral surgery ever practiced. Of the 388 sites on the body for use as an acupuncturist's pin cushion, twenty-six were for relief of toothache.

Cosmetic dentistry may have also been practiced. Marco Polo, in his best-seller *Travels*, published in 1295, wrote that in Karbandan in southern China, "Both the men and the women of this province have the custom of covering their teeth with thin plates of gold, which are fitted with great nicety to the shape of the teeth, and remain on them continually."

Japanese dental techniques were similar to China's, though when it came to curing a toothache, they were more apt to fight fire with fire, with moxibustion: Inflamed oral tissues were cauterized by igniting a moxa plant, or wads of cotton, wool, and other combustible substances, on the affected areas. Extractions were said to be performed using bare fingers in Japan; the procedure was practiced on wooden pegs driven into holes in boards.

Seeking Dental Nirvana

OVER THE JAGGED, razor-sharp teeth of the Himalayas, another dentally advanced culture developed between 4000 and 3000 B.C. This was the time of the appearance of the Vedas, the sacred Sanskrit writings of the ancient Hindus. The Agurveda, one of these texts, contains the history of Indian medicine and includes discourses on dentistry as well as the anatomy of the mouth, its pathology, treatment, and hygiene.

The toothworm also appears in these sacred texts, along with incantations against it similar to those recommended later in the Egyptian Papyrus Anastasi, dating from about 1000 B.C.

The Vishnu Veda, named for the supergod of the Hindu pantheon, devotes the entire sixty-first chapter to a detailed description of various ways to cleanse the teeth. The preferred tool, known as a Dantakashtha, was formed from a twig or small branch taken from any of various aromatic shrubs and frayed at the end. Careful attention was paid to the cleaning ritual.

Indian dental surgeons of the era treated patients for Upa Kusa (periodontitis to modern dentists, any degenerative condition of the bone holding the teeth in place, often accompanied by the discharge of purulent matter). Krimi-danta, as caries was known, were also treated and extractions performed. Tartar removal was another service. Jewelers specialized in ligating the teeth, tying loose ones to strong to hold them in place. Overall, extracting tools and other dental instruments of the era have been called "surprisingly modern in their construction."

In the time of Artreya—somewhere between the fifteenth century to the sixth century B.C.—Susruta Samhita was creating the eponymous *Susruta Samhita*, the monumental work that would become the basic text of Indian medicine. Susruta cataloged sixty-five diseases of the mouth and developed precise categories for each. An early advocate of oral hygiene, he echoed the Veda's admonition on brushing, advising "One should rise early in the morning and brush one's teeth. The tooth brush should consist of a fresh twig of a tree free from any knots, 12 fingers in length, and as thick as one's small finger."

Daily use of a cleansing paste made from honey, oil, and other ingredients was also recommended. He also described surgical instruments for various operations including forceps for extracting teeth.

The more one ponders India's divine dental heritage, the more the multiarmed deities of the holy Hindu pantheon suggest the four-handed dental procedures of modern dentists.

Holy Tooth

TODAY ON THE subcontinent, the tooth's primordial power and symbolism as a totem of life and object of veneration persists. It is embodied, or enameled, in the Sacred Tooth of Buddha, a religious treasure "that has caused endless wars and wanderings," in the words of Dr. Hermann Prinz, esteemed historian, scholar, and author of *Dental Chronology.*

The Perakara, one of the most closely guarded and holiest relics in the world, rests inside the innermost of seven silver caskets in the Dalada Maligarva—the Temple of the Tooth of Buddha—in Kandy, Sri Lanka, off the southern tip of India. Every month of Esala (July or August) during the "Festival of Elephants," it is taken from the temple and carried through the streets under a full moon in a grand procession 100 elephants long.

Early in the twentieth century, Sri Lanka, then Ceylon, was one of the ports of call on what was billed as the first round-the-world cruise open to the public. A dentist, H. L. Ambler, was on the voyage, and arranged to see the sacred relic. He recalled the tooth in *Around the World Dentistry,* a dentocentric account of the circumnavigation, describing it as "about three inches long and correspondingly thick. From our present knowledge of human anatomy we fail to see how any human being could have grown such a tooth."

An examination of the tooth's history explains the discrepancy. According to legend, the tooth was brought to the island in about 360 A.D. by Princess Kalinga, who spirited it out of India by hiding it in her hair, triggering more than a millennia of violence. One thousand years later, in 1315, Malabarsin succeeded in liberating the sacred relic and returned it to India. Not long after, Bahu Third stole it back.

The Portuguese gained possession of the tooth around 1500 when they conquered Ceylon. Determined to put a stop to the bloody clashes it had precipitated, they took it to Goa where it was burned by the archbishop in the presence of the viceroy and court. The powdered remains were then scattered in the sea.

Undeterred by the loss of his tooth, the khan, Wikrama Ahu, simply manufactured another from a piece of discolored ivory, making it some twenty times the size of a human tooth, and built the splendid palace where it now resides. Thus Dr. Ambler's assessment was correct: Not only isn't the sacred relic Buddha's tooth, it isn't even human, a well-known fact that has failed to stem the devotion of the devout.

A second putative tooth of Buddha belongs to China. On loan to Mynamar in 1996, it was displayed in the Kaba Aye temple, a Buddhist temple frequented by officials of the military regime. Thousand of pilgrims lined up daily to view the treasure. The Buddha's spirit of tranquil enlightenment was mocked when two bombs were set off in the temple. The government accused unknown perpetrators of trying to undermine ties with China, Mynamar's biggest arms supplier, by destroying the holy relic. Five people were killed. The tooth was unharmed.

The Roots of Western Dentistry

A DENTALLY ADVANCED civilization appeared in Italy during the first millennium before Christ. The signal event in its recognition was the development of artificial replacements for missing parts. In this case, the prosthetic appliances were dental bridges. The remnants of such a device found in Sidon, Lebanon, hint that seafaring Phoenicians may have been familiar with dental prostheses. But the first definitive evidence of their use was left by the Etruscans, citizens of Etruria, a small nation that occupied the hills of present-day Tuscany, from about 1000 to 400 B.C.

Predating neighboring Rome, little is known of this race. But from a dental standpoint they were highly advanced, creating fine bridges of gold rings and natural teeth that have been called "the greatest contributions to early prosthetic dental appliances." The bridges found in mouths around the world today are their descendants. A bridge is simply a replacement tooth or teeth mounted on a dental plate and, as the name implies, anchored to neighboring teeth for support.

Even the ancient Greeks didn't achieve this degree of restorative sophistication. When indisposed, early Greeks sought cures through magic and prayer, typically at temples dedicated to Aesculapius, god of medicine. Reputed to be the son of Apollo, there is confusion about the lineage of the medicine god. Cicero mentions three deities who shared this name. One was said to have been the son of Arsippus, the god who taught the world tooth-drawing and bloodletting. A flesh-and-blood Aesculapius, the chief of Thessaly, is described by Homer in the Odyssey as a skillful surgeon who, with godlike hands, helped wounded Greeks at the walls of Troy.

As time elapsed, more gods became known as Aesculapius and more temples for the sick and infirm were built in their name. The Western tradition of dentistry began as one of the healing arts practiced at these temples. Among the most renown Aesculapian temples was that of Kos. Here, in the first year of the eightieth Olympiad, 460 B.C., Hippocrates, the Western world's Father of Medicine, was born. It was at this shrine to superstition, magic, and quackery that Hippocrates gained the majority of his medical knowledge—most of which he promptly renounced.

Claiming kinship with Aesculapius of Thessaly (the seventeenth descendant by some accounts), Hippocrates preached that medicine should be disassociated from magic and priestcraft, commencing the West's first steps toward the secularization of medicine. Rejecting the primitive notion that spirits caused illness, Hippocrates embraced the humoral theory, stating that the four fluids of the body were the primary elements of both health and disease. Pneumatic theories added the principles of heat, cold, wetness, and dryness to humoral concepts, enabling the cause of some disorders to be properly identified: engorgement by blood. It was to control these humors and the resulting ill health that bloodletting became a standard medical practice, one which survived into the twentieth century.

His doctrine led to the gradual abandonment of Aesculapian temples in favor of medical "shops," each specializing in selected ailments. Soon the shops sprang up everywhere and flocks of diseased and infirm followed. It may have been within one of these shops that dentistry had its birth as an independent medical practice in the West.

Hippocrates attached great importance to diseases of the dental system and wrote extensively about maladies of the teeth and gums. Tooth decay, he believed, was caused in part by individual predisposition and in part by the corrosive action of food and debris trapped around already weakened teeth. He recommended using cautery and astringents to remove the morbid humors that resulted. He also invented crude dental forceps for extractions and other dental instruments.

The Greeks' practice of tooth extractions represents a step forward in the dental arts, though the name of the instrument employed sounds like a monster from an Odyssean journey: the odontagogon, or plumbeum odontagogon. The ultimate example of the tool reputedly hung in the Temple of Apollo at Delphi. Resembling an oversize pair of forceps, its malleable lead (plumbeum) construction has been said by some to reflect the Greeks' belief that only teeth loose enough to be plucked by such a soft metal should be extracted. (Hippocrates advised leaving the tooth in place if the odontagogon couldn't dislodge it.) However, it is likely that the odontogogon of Delphi was a model, upon which smaller forceps made of harder metal would be based.

Hippocrates' description of a tooth extraction using the plumbeum odontagogon is said by some to be the first dental operation referred to in historical records. He also pondered connections between the mouth, physiognomy, and health.

"Among those individuals whose heads are long in shape," he wrote, "some have thick necks . . . others have strongly arched palates, their teeth disposed irregularly, crowding one on the other and they are molested by headaches and otorrhea."

However, Hippocrates' dental writings contain critical errors. He believed men had more teeth than women, revealing, as one historian noted, that he "failed to make personal explorative simple examinations, like looking inside the mouth."

Aristotle (384–322 B.C.) included teeth in his investigation of self and universe. Founder of the study of comparative anatomy, he devoted an entire chapter to the subject in *De partibus animalium* (Parts of Animals). It contained the first scientific study of the oral organs, though as the title suggests, the teeth were animal (pig) rather than human. Aristotle described the blood supply of the teeth as well as the extraction process. As part of this latter subject, he addressed the mechanics of the forceps *(sideros)*, pointing out the advantage of "two levers, acting in contrary sense having a single fulcrum." This was written a 100 years before the principle of the lever was set down; thus, the teeth can claim credit for inspiring the first explanation of the workings of this simple machine a century before Archimedes received credit for it. Not so impressive is the fact that like Hippocrates, Aristotle believed men had more teeth than women.

Dentus Maximus

THE GLORY OF Rome was reflected in the mouths of its leading citizens, whose dental work and prostheses marked the zenith of the ancient world's oral-care arts. Famous for their feats of building roads, bridges, and grand edifices, Romans were equally skilled at construction within the confines of the oral cavity. They invented gold shell crowns, new methods of securing loose teeth, and created artificial replacements in a selection of materials including bone, boxwood, and ivory.

Numerous examples of Roman dental work have survived, though their owners were often cremated. It was customary to remove prosthetic devices before bodies were burned, and return the appliance to the ashes for internment afterward. This was perceived as a waste by officials, as gold was used to make these devices and Rome was eager to protect its supply of the precious metal. This was one of the issues addressed when demands for a written code of rules resulted in the enactment of Rome's first laws in 450 B.C., the Law of the XII Tables. Among the rules: "Neither shall gold be added thereto (to the corpse); but it shall not be unlawful to bury or burn it (the corpse) with the gold with which the teeth may be perchance be bound together." In other words, gold that had been permanently affixed to the teeth could be left in place; there was no need to desecrate the body. But any removable dental appliances with gold had to be taken out before cremation and burial. The code also set penalties for knocking out the teeth of either a freeman or a slave. These laws represent Rome's first record of dentistry.

By the first century A.D., a prospective Roman dental patient could choose a physician specializing in dentistry, a tooth-drawer or barber-surgeon. There was plenty of work to go around for these practitioners. Had Marc Antony asked to borrow his countrymen's teeth rather than their ears, he would have seen that caries and dental infections of all kinds were rampant in Rome. The first urine of the morning was advised as a medicinal mouthwash and the urine of young boys was considered best. One historian suggested that "little fellows paid for such substances may be ancestors of today's dentists."

Like the Greeks, Romans practiced extractions. Their instrument of choice, a *dentiducem*, was based on the odontogogon design. Tooth-drawers specialized in these procedures, while barber-surgeons cornered the market in bloodletting and leaching, as well as cupping and cosmetic shaping of teeth, all treatments considered beneath a physician. Cupping, a humoral-based therapy, involved drawing blood to the skin with a suction apparatus, typically a hot cup pressed against the flesh and allowed to cool.

In the first half of the first century A.D., the first cavity is believed to have been filled. Aulus Cornelius Celsus (25 B.C.–A.D. 50) performed the procedure. His fillings of lint and lead were often put in place only to give his forceps something to grip and prevent a tooth from shattering during an extraction.

A physician and encyclopedist, Celsus wrote widely on dental subjects. He believed toothaches and abscesses "may be numbered among the worst of tortures," and recommended a narcotic cocktail for respite, prepared from cinnamon, mandrake, opium poppy, and castoreum. His only surviving work, *De re medicina,* in eight volumes, contains detailed descriptions and accounts of the treatment of dental disease. Though it was not printed until 1478, by the midpoint of the twentieth century, the book was still said to have had more editions to its credit than any other medical volume written.

Celsus saw oral health as a reflection of overall wellness. "If a gangrene seizes ulcers of the mouth," he wrote, "it must be considered in the first place whether the body be in a bad habit; if it be, that must be rectified, and then must proceed to the cure of the ulcers."

For the cure, weak vinegar and astringents, and chewing unripe pears and apples were among his recommendations. The alternative therapy was less pleasant: "When this latter however cannot be obtained by drugs, the ulcer must be cauterized with a red hot iron." Applications of arsenic were also part of the protocol.

For extractions, Celsus advised completely detaching the gum around the tooth, a painful proposition in the days before anesthesia. The tooth was then digitally manipulated until loose enough to yank out, by the fingers or with a slender-beaked forceps the Greeks had developed called a "rhizagra." Heavy bleeding in the aftermath of the procedure was an indication that some part of the jawbone had been broken. Bone fragments resulting from such mistakes had to be removed, typically be cutting a large incision in the gum for access. According to Celsus, recovery usually began within fourteen to twenty-one days of the procedure.

The Toothworm Moves West

IT WAS DURING this time—about A.D. 41—that the toothworm made its official entrance into Western dental literature, imported by Scribonius Largus in *De compositione medicamentorum,* the first medical formulary of the Western world. Largus passed along the accepted wisdom that toothworms caused decay and toothaches. The belief would survive in mainstream Western dental theory well into the Middle Ages and among the masses for far longer.

Largus also recorded the standard cure of the time: burn seeds of hyoscyamus, or henbane—the dried leaves of the plant *Hyoscyamus niger*—on charcoal and inhale the fumes. The fumes would cause the worms to fall from the teeth. Not coincidentally, henbane is a narcotic. The vapor no doubt soothed and relieved the pain, and the soporific effect probably helped blur the fact that seedbuds of henbane, when burned, leave an ash resembling worms. This residue was offered as proof to centuries of sufferers of both the toothworms' existence and the efficacy of this method of removal.

Largus was the first to describe the preparation of opium from poppy heads, as well. Dentist to Emperor Claudius, he also left a record of the dental hygiene practices of Mesalina, Claudius's infamous wife known for her voracious sexual appetite. Her tooth powder, Largus claimed, was made of mastic of chios, sal ammoniac (a chloride of ammonia), and calcined stags' horn. Though no doubt added for its abrasive properties, can this last ingredient, long reputed as an aphrodisiac, help explain Mesalina's predilection for wanton libidinal adventures? If so, then historians must add dentifrice to the causative factors in the empire's moral, if not oral decay.

A wealth of misinformation was added to Western dental theory by Gaius Plinius Secundus, Pliny the Elder (A.D. 23–79), the encyclopedist and fabulist historian. It is easy in hindsight to question the accuracy of his accounts, but at the time reports like the following, which Pliny quoted, may have seemed plausible:

> In many mountains of India . . . there are men with dogs' heads who clothe themselves with skins and bark instead of speaking; also men having only one leg, who have great speed in leaping, and others without any neck who have their eyes between their shoulders.

Of the 160 volumes he wrote, only *Historia naturalis*, a natural history encyclopedia in thirty-seven books, remains. Among the wisdom that can be found in its pages:

In the teeth of man there exists a poisonous substance which has the effect of dimming the brightness of a looking glass when they are presented uncovered before it and if they are uncovered in front of young unfledged pigeons, these take ill and die.

In the fullers thistle, a herb which grows near the rivers, is found a small worm which has the power of curing dental pains, when the said worm is killed by rubbing it on the teeth, or when it is closed up with wax in hollow teeth.

Pliny suggested that if the first tooth to fall out did not touch the ground, it could keep a woman's private parts pain-free if mounted on a bracelet and worn at all times. Like the learned Greeks before him, he believed "Men have thirty-two teeth, women a lesser number, and to have a greater number than usual is considered an indication of long life."

Folk-medicine cures, which Pliny recorded and ascribed to, included a remedy for painful gums that called for scratching the affected area with the tooth of a man who met a violent death. And loose teeth, he wrote, could be made firm with a whole frog tied to the jaw. For prevention of toothache, he suggested eating a mouse twice a month. If a toothache was already present, "bite on a piece of wood from a tree struck by lightning," or "touch the tooth with the frontal bone of a lizard taken during the full moon." Juice extracted from plants grown inside the human skull were also high on his list of palliatives.

As one historian pointed out, "Dental quacks of those days probably misrepresented, selling wood which hadn't really been hit by lightning, bones of lizards caught during other moon phases, and extracts of plants grown in skulls of any animals they could find."

An Eye for a Lie and a Tooth for a Truth

GIVEN THE WIDESPREAD ignorance and gullibility that Pliny's writings suggest, belief in spirits and demons as agents of infirmity remained strong. Telling a lie, for example, was thought to invite immediate retribution from the gods in the form of an injury or loss of a tooth, eye, or other body part. Horace, the first-century poet, alluded to this belief as well as a man's ability to be blinded by beauty to such obvious signs of fecklessness in his ode "To Barine":

If E'er th' insulted powers had shed
Their vengeance on thy perjured head;
If they had marked thy faithless troth
With one foul nail, or blacken'd tooth
Again thy falsehood might deceive
And I the faithless vow believe.

Despite the persistence of superstition and ignorance, dentistry was making progress. Near the end of the first century, Archigenes (A.D. 81–117), a Syrian who was among the elite of Roman surgeons and physicians, asserted that in some cases toothaches resulted from disease occurring in the interior of the tooth, in its root. When pained patients appeared with a discolored tooth resistant to the usual remedies, he applied a trephine, a cylindrical saw for cutting through bone he invented, and bored through the tooth to the pulp chamber to release the morbid humors, or "accumulated pus" as a more modern dental writer termed it.

Galen (Claudius Galenus, A.D. 129–201), among the most famous and acclaimed men of medicine in Rome, attributed toothaches to "the internal action of acrid and corroding humors, that is, it is produced in the same manner as those cutaneous ulcers which appear without any influence or external cause."

This put Galen squarely in the humorist camp. Born at Pergamum in Asia Minor and educated in Alexandria, Galen is remembered today as one of antiquity's most gifted students of the natural sciences. He is said to have given us the dental nomenclature of incisors and was the first to recognize nerves (pulps) in the teeth.

Though a gifted anatomist, he was off the mark on some of his dental theories. He classified teeth and bones, believed they were involved in the sense of taste, and thought they could grow and repair themselves through a regenerative nutritional process. His therapeutic recommendations are also open to question. To relieve a toothache, he advised rubbing the gums with the milk of a bitch or the brains of a hare. If a tooth protruded above the level of the others, he advised filing it down, without regard to the fit with its opposite tooth above or below.

Another of Rome's famed physicians, Paul of Aigina, also put his mind where his mouth was. Seven volumes of his book *On Medicine* detail his beliefs. Oral health received attention commencing with the first tome:

The teeth will not decay if the following things be attended to; in the first place avoid indigestion and frequent repetition of emetics.

Guard against such food as is hurtful to the teeth, dried figs, honey boiled so as to become very hard, dates, and all glutinous substances . . . The teeth ought to be cleaned after supper.

Paul also addressed the problem of teething pain. He recommended digitally massaging a youngster's gums for relief. The choice of salves he recommended—either fat of fowl or the brain of a hare—provided enough dietal variety so that even today one or the other are usually available to most households.

Yet while dentistry was advancing, the empire was decaying. The dental glory that was Rome, the minimonuments to vanity and oral utility, would disappear with its fall, and the Dark Ages that followed cast a pall over oral health for the next thousand years.

2

From Swindling Charlatans to Bleeding Barbers

The Incompetence of Tooth-Drawers Is Equalled by the Barbarity of Barber-Surgeons

A TRUMPET BLARES, CALLING THE RABBLE TO GATHER BEFORE A stage in the marketplace. On the raised platform, a chattering monkey surveys the throng from beneath a parasol while a juggler performs tricks and recites ribald jokes, warming up the assembly. Now the juggler retires, the music stops, and a commanding figure bolts onto the stage dressed in a magnificent plumed hat and rich tunic, a necklace of human teeth strung about his neck. Soon his boastful oration has lured a recalcitrant toothache sufferer to the stage. It is over in a moment. The troublesome tooth is out, quickly and painlessly. The volunteer looks on, stunned, as the tooth-drawer holds the tooth aloft for the crowd's delectation. Now more of the orally afflicted press forward to submit to the tooth-drawer's ministrations. It is unlikely those lining up will have as unpainful an experience as the confederate who just pretended to have his tooth drawn. But the blare of horn and beating of drum will drown out their cries. And by the time sepsis sets in or other life-threatening complications arising from the tooth-drawer's incompetence present themselves, the charlatan will be long gone.

This is the dentist's office of the Middle Ages. To be sure, there were alternatives. The sufferer could avail himself to a barber-surgeon—either for an extraction or to be bled in lieu of such an invasive procedure—or he could choose from a multitude of the useless elixirs that promised quick relief from all dental discomfort. But the reputable physicians who'd dabbled in dentistry in Roman times had fled the field with the fall of the empire, leaving what we consider dentistry to these incompetents, ignoramuses, quacks, and charlatans.

Physicians' reluctance to practice dentistry was understandable; medicine was extremely limited in its ability to alleviate dental pain or treat its cause. Despite the pontificating by Hippocrates and his peers, oral care was considered slumming by many antiquarian health-care professionals, an attitude that persisted through the Middle Ages. As late as the 1500s, Swiss professor of medicine Theodor Zwinger advised physicians against performing tooth extractions, saying it was best left to barbers and charlatans, as the operation was fraught with "unpleasant accidents" including fractured jaws, lacerated gums, and serious hemorrhaging. Celebrated Dutch physician Kornelis Van Soolingen spoke contemptuously of dental operations more than a century later.

Alternative Treatments

AS PHYSICIANS HAD good reason to turn their backs on dentistry, the public had good reason to do the same to tooth-drawers and their brethren. They were regarded as practitioners of last resort, owing to the pain and danger inherent in their treatments. People with toothaches would do almost anything to avoid submitting to them, a desperation that drove the thriving market in worthless or dangerous potions, tinctures, and salves. The growth of this trade was marked by the opening of England's first apothecary in 1345. One cannot help but wonder what the grand-opening event was like in a far less media-saturated age.

We can assume the inventory included palliatives for oral afflictions. In the toothworm section, one would expect to find the popular remedies of the Medieval era: honey, bitter plants, myrrh, aloe, colocynth, and acids like the gastric juice of pigs.

A thirteenth-century manuscript, *Leechdoms, Wortcunning and Starcraft* (roughly translated into modern English as "Medicine, Natural Remedies and Astrology") contained many references to dental disease and a collection of folk remedies for toothaches, echoing the disinformation spread by quacks of yore.

> For tooth-worms take acorn-meal and henbane-seed and wax,
> of all equally much. Mix them together. Make them into a wax

candle, and burn it; let it reek into the mouth, put a black cloth under, then shall the worms fall on it.

For tooth wark: if a worm eat the tooth, take an old hollylead, hartwort, and sage. Boil in water, pour it into a bowl, and yawn over it; then the worms shall fall into the bowl.

For tooth wark, fray to dust the rind of nut tree and thorntree; cut the teeth on the outside, shed the dust on frequently. For the upper toothache take leaves of withe, wind and wring them on the nose. For the nether toothache, slit the gums with the instrument till they bleed.

If the tooth had to go, advice on painless extractions was also rendered:

Take some newts, by some called lizards, and those nasty beetles which are found in ferns in the summer time. Calcine them in an iron pot, and make a powder thereof. Wet the forefinger of the right hand, and insert it in the powder, and apply it to the tooth frequently, refraining from spitting it off, when the tooth will fall away without pain. It is proven.

A fifteenth-century "leechbook," an instructional tome on the application of leeches, proffered similar therapies, such as the one "For aching of the hollow tooth":

Take raven's dung and put it in the hollow tooth and colour it with the juice of pellitory of Spain that the sick recognize it not nor know what it be; and then put it in the tooth and it shall break the tooth and take away the aching as some men say, it will make the tooth fall out.

If none of these remedies worked, there were a host of medical procedures for treating toothache that stopped well short of extractions. Accepted therapies included blood-letting, leeching, blistering of the skin, laxatives, cupping, placing garlic cloves in the ear, and destroying the dental nerves by cautery using a red-hot iron or strong acid.

By the time one was ready and willing to submit to a tooth-drawer, he was probably in terrible agony and a tooth most surely had to be extracted. Whether it would be the right one, and whether the exractee would survive was open to question.

Naming Names

IN ROMAN TIMES roving tooth-drawers were called *dentatores, dentispices,* or *edentarii.* During the Middle Ages they practiced throughout Europe, changing their methods little over the centuries.

Itinerant tooth-drawers traversed the English countryside, where they also went by the name of toothers, toothis, and, of all things, kind-hearts. They were called *cavadenti* in Italy, *arracheurs de dents* in France, and *zahnbrecher* or *tenebreker* in Germany. But that barely touches the surface of the name-calling associated with its practitioners. Arguably history's most excoriated health-care providers, tooth-drawers earned an enmity reflected in the many synonyms applied to them. Among the common terms were charlatan, quack-doctor, quack-salver, quack, mountebank, empiric, *saltinbancoe,* pretender, and counterfeit physician. These designations echo through the pages of dental history.

The word charlatan comes from Italian *ciarlatano,* which means one who sells salves and other drugs in public places, pulls teeth, and exhibits tricks or legerdemain. Its root, the noun *ciarla,* means empty garrulity and the verb *ciarlare* means to speak in a boastful and irresponsible fashion, frequently with the intention of confusing others.

The Dutch suggest that their term for quack-salver, *Kwabzalver,* comes from *kwab,* a sebaceous cyst or wen, and *zalver,* an ointment; many quacks probably offered to cure cysts and wens with their potions. Germans said it came from *quecksilber,* a Teutonic version of quicksilver (metallic mercury), a substance used widely in both medicine and quackery.

The first mention of quacks in English literature appeared in *Schoole of Abuse,* printed in 1579, which referred to "A quacke-saluer's Budget of filthy receites." The term *quack* may be a shortened form of quack-salver, a seller of ointments. Or it may also be a derivative of quake, the fevers; the doctors who cured them—or tried to—were called quake doctors. *The Oxford Dictionary* offered this definition: "An ignorant pretender to medical and surgical skill, who boasts to have a knowledge of wonderful remedies, an empiric, an imposter in medicine." *Samuel Johnson's Dictionary*, written in 1755, defined quack as: "1. A boastful pretender to arts which he does not understand; 2. A vain, boastful pretender to physic, one who proclaims his own medical abilities in public places; 3. An artful, tricking practitioner in physic."

Others suggest that quack may come from the sound it is associated with in English: that of ducks, implying noisome and meaningless talk. Skeats's *Etymological Dictionary of the English Language* defines quack as "to cry out pretended nostrums" as well as "to make a noise like a duck," and notes that "the word originally meant a mountebank who sold salves and eye lotions at country fairs."

A mountebank originally referred to a tooth-drawer who performed his craft while astride a horse, a flamboyant and dangerous practice performed in England and Italy. It came to refer to a traveling quack who, prior to conducting business, regaled an audience and potential patients from a stage, telling stories, performing tricks, and juggling. The mountebank was often seconded by an assistant dressed in the costume of a clown or harlequin, including the pointed cap of the fool. The assistant was called, among other names, a zany, *factotum*, or Merry Andrew. This last nickname is believed to have been taken from Dr. Andrew Borde, a physician to Henry VIII noted for his wit and humor.

Dirty Drawers

THE TRADEMARK OF the itinerant tooth-drawer was a banner and parasol. A small alligator hung from the parasol, according to some accounts, signifying the piece of "alligator tail" stuffed in the empty tooth socket following extraction to staunch the bleeding. Pointed hats bearing the insignia of St. Apollonia, patron saint of toothache sufferers, and a necklace of extracted human teeth were also part of their standard regalia.

They performed their craft, or skullduggery, out of doors, for they required light. Crowds were also important, both to increase the pool of potential patients and to create the excitement that stimulated business. Fairs, marketplaces, and bazaars were prime sites for their theatrics, which was essentially entertainment, or performance art. Over time, more pageantry was added to these events. The operating platform evolved into an elaborate stage. The tooth-drawer spent less time warming up the crowd, turning the duties over to professional entertainers. Songs and other presurgery amusements would start the show. Clowns, conjurers, and jugglers were among the entertainers employed to draw crowds. When the tooth-drawer—often an inept charlatan—took the stage, he customarily described his credentials, typically all fatuous and invented.

Tooth-drawers left almost no written records of their own, but we know something of their MO from paintings and artwork. The earliest engraving of such a subject, created by Lucas van Leyden of the Netherlands in 1523, shows the toothpuller studiously engaged in removing a tooth from the patient's mouth. A female accomplice is meanwhile engaged in picking the patient's purse.

Between 1600 and 1700, tooth-drawers were the subjects of canvases by several major artists. Jan Steen, Jan J. van Vliet, Rombouts, and other Dutch and Flemish masters painted itinerant toothpullers at work in towns and villages, providing captivating depictions of their operations and the period. The pomp, pageantry, and pain is captured in the full range, from the lone, hardscrabble tooth-drawer, to the staged performances of the era's successful charlatans.

Not all tooth-drawers were crooks and deceivers. Some were merely incompetent. Others may have been fairly adept at their craft, but without modern equipment or painkillers, treatment, no matter how competent, was assuredly a horrific experience. Looking back in history, distinguishing between the honest blunderer and the outright quack is as difficult now as it was then.

For example, empiric or empirical pretender is considered synonymous with quack by some, whereas others contend they represented a distinct class that specialized in experimental remedies. The term empiric is said to come from an ancient sect of physicians who disregarded theoretical study, basing their knowledge on practical experience.

Contemptible Infamy

JOURNEYMAN TOOTH-DRAWERS LED a rough life. They had to compete for business with barber-surgeons and the out-and-out charlatans, who had no compunctions about making the boldest claims for their skills.

Some performed bloodletting, bonesetting, and corn-cutting on the feet to augment their income. The first identified, England's William le Tothdrawer, resorted to deception and assault to supplement his meager earnings. Imprisoned, he was said to have been subsequently released due to poverty—and this was in a country that maintained jails for debtors, a reflection, perhaps, of society's regard for his profession as beneath contempt.

In 1595 Henry Chettle, a London dramatist and bookseller, published a pamphlet, "Kind-heart's Dreame," describing the life of an itinerant tooth-drawer of the period. From this work the term *kind heart* came to be considered synonymous with tooth-drawer, though it's unclear if the kind heart of the title was an individual or a generic term for the trade. The attire he described was typical enough of the time, a costume that included a string of extracted teeth on his belt and a woolen cap with a large leaden brooch adorned with an effigy of St. George. He addressed readers thusly:

> Gentlemen and good fellows, whose kindness having christened me with the name of Kind heart, binds me in all kind course I can to deserve the continuance of your love, let it seem not strange, I beseech you, that he that all his life hath been famous for drawing teeth should now in drooping age hazard contemptible infamy by drawing himself into print.

The class had already achieved contemptible infamy many times over. *The Anatomies of the True Physician and Counterfeit Mountebank*, written in 1605, provides a glimpse of the breadth of those offering their services as tooth-drawers and healers, and the regard in which they were held.

> The whole Rable of these quack-Saluers are of a base wit and perverse. They for the most part are the abject and sordidous scumme and refuse of the people, who having run away from their trades and occupations leane in a corner to get their livings by killing men, and if we . . . bring them to the light, which like owls they cannot abide, they will appear to be runagate Jews, the cut-throats and robbers of Christians, slow-bellied monks who had made escape from their cloisters, Simoniacal and perjured shavelings, busy St. John-lack-Latins, thrasonical

and unlettered chemists, shifting and outcast pettifoggers, light-headed and trivial druggers and apothecaries, sun-shunning night-birds and corner creepers, dull-pated and base mechanics, stage players, jugglers, pedlars, prittle-prattling barbers, filthy graziers, curious bathkeepers, common shifters and cogging cavaliers, bragging soldiers, lazy clowns, one-eyed and lamed fencers, toothless and tattling old wives, chattering charwomen and nurse-keepers, scape-Tyburns, dog-leeches and suchlike baggage.

And those, according to the book, were the better ones.

In the next rank, to second this goodly troupe, follow poisoners, enchanters, wizards, fortune tellers, magicians, witches and hags.

If one thing can be said for tooth-drawers, they were often leaders of the packs of riffraff with whom they traveled. Court masques and other popular dramatic presentations of the era sometimes referred to them. In one production, "Pan's Anniversary," a group of country bumpkins is led by a tooth-drawer. "A tooth-drawer is our foreman," avers a member of the motley crew. "Hee draws teeth a horse-backe in full speed."

Itinerant tooth-drawers of seventeenth century Scotland likewise led a lively crowd, according to the following account by J. Menzies Campbell:

A horde of arrogant mountebanks whose policy was never that of self-abnegation, systematically traveled around the country, their visits coinciding with local markets and fairs . . . They glibly promised cures for every disease including toothache. There was always a zany who, in a droll manner, sang lewd yet amusing songs riveting the attention of disorders which his master could cure.

The entourage also included dancers with curious antics and performers on the tight rope. The bedizened quicksilver enliv-ened the proceedings with comic orations, while perched on a well-appointed chariot drawn by four (sometimes six) elegantly caparisoned horses. Not infrequently, he reinforced his claims by quoting scripture or by prayers to saints. Although never averse to superstitious cases which he had miraculously cured, he remained profoundly silent on the array of persons he had caused to suffer grievously or even liquidated. Tooth-drawing was always one of the most popular sidelines to entertain the crowd of ignoramuses, who besieged his stage.

Not all quacks practiced dentistry, but those that did often cut particularly memorable figures. Martin van Butchell, a small, bizarre bearded dental quack who armed himself with a white bone, rode about London on a white pony painted with purple spots. After his wife died, van Butchell had her embalmed and kept in his house in a glass case, making sure to introduce all his guests to her. The crowds that resulted necessitated the following notice in the *St. James Chronicle* in 1775:

> Van Butchell (not willing to be unpleasantly circumstanced, and wishing to convince some good minds they have been misinformed) acquaints the Curious, no stranger can see his embalmed Wife, unless (by a Friend personally) introduced to himself, anyday between Nine and One, Sundays excepted.

David Perronet, another Londoner, specialized in bloodletting and treating toothaches, which he promised to cure with his "Universal dentifrice" which made "black teeth as ivory, and a sure and speedy remedy for the worst Teethaches from such as be hollow and rotten; for be they never so raging or of long continued, this remedy will presently cure it by Killing the Worm in it."

If Perronet's dentifrice failed to control the worms, consumers could try the *Pulvis Benedictus*, or Worm Exterminator, a potion that took a book of fifteen chapters to explain its powers. The book told of "Mr. Stiles of the Lock and Key in West-Smithfield, who was practically eaten by a worm 8 feet long, and might still have been alive, if he had only taken the Exterminator, which is looked upon to be rather a miracle than a medicine."

C. J. S. Thompson, in *The Quacks of Old London*, noted "England was the quack's Eldorado; and they flocked to London from all parts of Europe ready to cure every imaginable ill." The opportunity for fame and fortune was great, if one was quick-witted and without scruples. But the training was rigorous. An account quoted in Thompson's book details the education of the seventeenth-century quack doctor William Salmon:

> When a boy [Salmon] was apprenticed to a mountebank whom he served as a "wachum" or "zany," and used to inveigh and direct the amazed silly rout, with tumbling through a hoop and vaulting and amusing them with tricks and legerdemain and sleight of hand. He served him also as Juggler, Sub-conjurer, Astrologer, ganymede and orator; made speeches and wrote Panygyricks in praise of his master's Panaceas. He wrote Almanacks to direct the taking of his medicines, and made the stars vouch for their virtue. He calculated nativities, told fortunes, had admirable secrets to the Sodderacked Maidenheads, and Incomparable Philters for the consolation of despairing Damsels.

After graduating to being a quack himself, Salmon amassed a fortune selling worthless remedies.

Quack à la Mode

IN FRANCE, THE Pont-Neuf bridge in Paris was a crossroads of quackery from the seventeenth to nineteenth centuries. Here, medical and dental charlatans of all stripes gathered. One of the most renowned was Le Grand Thomas, an immense man who "ate for four, drank in the same proportions, and slept eighteen hours out of twenty-four." An eighteen-century print depicts him garbed in a three-cornered hat with a plume of peacock feathers and a scarlet coat braided in gold. A fancy dagger was strapped to his side, the emblem of a shining sun over his heart and around his neck a chain of teeth.

By the eighteenth century in France, the tooth-drawer's repute had passed into the vernacular in the popular adage of the time, *Mentir comme un aracheur de dents*, or "lie like a tooth drawer."

Pierre Fauchard, who would earn acclaim as the Father of Dentistry, referred to the Pont-Neuf scene as the "Theater of impostors." He also explained how these tooth-drawers hoodwinked the public:

If there are secrets for drawing the teeth with so much facility
as the operators of the market place and the public places try
to persuade the people, I admit they cannot be paid too much,
since they spare so much pain to those who have the misfortune
to be attacked by toothache and to be violently tormented by
it. The knowledge that I have of the teeth and the disease which
attack them has always convinced me that these kinds of people
have only one method, by throwing dust in people's eyes. The
trouble I have taken to discover the mystery of these impostors
has shown me and put me in possession of their cheat. All their
cleverness consists in getting hold of some unfortunates, who
push themselves among the people listening to the promises of
the empiric. These pretended paid sufferers come up from time
to time to the operator who holds in his hand a tooth all ready
wrapped in a very fine skin with blood of a chicken or some
other animal, introduces his hand in the mouth of the pretended
sufferer, drops into it the tooth hidden in his hand. Then he
has only to touch the tooth or do something of the sort with a
powder or a straw or the point of his sword, he has only if he
wishes to ring a bell in the ear of the pretended patient, who
spits during this time that which he has in his mouth. One sees
him spit out blood and the bloody tooth, which is only the tooth
which the impostor or the patient has introduced into the
mouth.

Once the ruse had been accomplished, the tooth-drawer was free
to yank anyone else's teeth without regard to the pain he caused. The
cacophony of the boisterous, incited crowd would typically drown out
any cries. If it appeared too difficult to extract for whatever reason, the
tooth-drawer might explain that the it was an eyetooth, and pulling it
would result in loss of the eye. Since antiquity, folk wisdom had held
that eyeteeth—the upper incisors and canines—and eyes were connected, which was another example of ignorance Fauchard railed
against:

If these impostors had learnt that part of surgery which they
debase by their impudent practice and gross ignorance, if they
had studied anatomy, they would know that the nerves which
go to the canines come from the same source as those of the

other teeth, and that the eye has no more connection with the teeth which they call eyeteeth than with the others.

There are as many eyeteeth for these pretended dentists as there are teeth in the mouth, for whenever they meet those which appear to them difficult to draw, they sheathe their sword quickly, with the point of which they boasted they drew them and thus put into the scabbard all the adroit blows of which they make parade, in the provinces and in Paris on the Pont-Neuf, the usual theater of these impostors, who having alarmed the sufferers by this and also the notion of eyeteeth, assure them after that, that, except for a certain sum, they cannot cure them, and that they have for their ache a grand infallible remedy of which they alone possess the secret. The sufferers, who are weak enough to believe them, find themselves duped by their audacious practice as well as by their bad theory.

Extracting Revenge

PAINLESS EXTRACTIONS WERE counterproductive when the tooth was being extracted for punitive purposes. Religious heretics and common criminals were among those sometimes sentenced to lose one or more teeth. The total was determined by the severity of the offense. Eating flesh on Lent joined a list of felonies sufficiently heinous to warrant one or more teeth being remanded for removal.

The upper incisor and canine—eyeteeth—were typically the first choice, possibly because of ease of access at the front of the mouth and the dramatic visual impact created by their absence. Among the criminal class, the trade-off between possible illicit gain and potential tooth loss was always at the top of their minds when planning a caper. Thus, objects of great desire ultimately were referred to as things for which one would gladly give an eyetooth.

England's King John (1167–1216), noted for brutality and lack of ethics, extorted 10,000 ducats from a rich Bristol man by confining him to his palace and personally pulling a tooth a day for seven days until finally his subject capitulated.

If it seems barbaric for the church to be involved in punitive extractions, perhaps the practice can be ascribed as a payback for a cruelty inflicted on one of their own—St. Apollonia, patron saint of toothache sufferers and the orally afflicted faithful everywhere.

St. Apollonia

IT'S NOT CONSIDERED polite to find comfort in the misfortune of others, but for more than 1,500 years, God-fearing toothache sufferers have been doing just that, thanks to the beneficence and sacrifice of the Christian martyr Apollonia. No one personifies their woes and suffering better than she. One unmindful of charges of sacrilege might suggest that what Christ did for mankind's sins, she did for his toothaches.

Apollonia was born in Alexandria, Egypt, daughter of a "heathen magistrate," as history recalls him, about two-and-a-half centuries after the death of Christ. It was a time when the word of Jesus challenged that of the pagan deities. According to legend, before Apollonia's birth, her mother was sympathetic to the Christians, though not a believer herself. Childless and desperate, she prayed to the Virgin for a baby. As Apollonia, the resulting miracle tot grew, her mother inculcated her with stories of the wondrous power of prayer. These tales must have had a dramatic impact, for young Apollonia became a disciple of St. Anthony of Egypt and was baptized by St. Leonine. Told to go forth and preach the Word, she took to the streets of Alexandria, her passionate preaching claiming many a convert.

Unfortunately, a backlash against the Christians was building. In A.D. 249, Christians were persecuted in Alexandria and set upon by mobs. Apollonia's teachings became a lightning rod for complaints. The matter was brought before her father. Perhaps weary himself from her tireless prostheletizing, he promptly handed her up to the governor for judgment.

Brought before the idol temple and ordered to worship the graven image, Apollonia reportedly made the sign of the cross, provoking an angry evil spirit to issue from the idol. In an effort to secure her compliance, her teeth were broken and extracted, one by one. (Punitive extractions were a common torture of the Roman Empire, as was crucifixion.) Still she refused to yield. When no teeth remained, officials clubbed her about the head and face. Given one more chance to recant, Apollonia jumped of her own volition into a fire. She is said to have prayed before her immolation that those remembering her pain and suffering in their prayers might themselves never have a toothache. Her fiery leap of faith has been a source of comfort, solace, and relief to the faithful almost ever since.

Canonized by the Church of Rome in A.D. 300, February 9 is celebrated as her day of commemoration. Her intercession is sought for relief of dental pains of all manner. One of many prayers to her:

O holy Apollonia, intercede for us by thy passion, by thy suffering in the teeth, throat and tongue, that we may be delivered from pain in the teeth now and for ever.

Apollonia's name was also invoked by quacks specializing in teething and toothache cures. During the fifteenth century a cure had to have a saint's name attached to be considered effective, and Apollonia's was more popular than any other. Religious relics said to be the bones of Apollonia were also believed to possess miraculous healing and curative powers for oral afflictions. Her teeth were considered the most powerful of her remaining parts in preventing toothache. King Henry VI, a deeply religious man, was so appalled at the widespread use and belief in these relics that he ordered all of them turned over to his agents. According to accounts of the roundup, "a ton of veritable teeth of St. Apollonia were thus collected together, and were her stomach proportionate to her teeth, a country could scarce afford her a meal."

Today, bits are what are said to be Apollonia's remains are housed in reliquaries from Antwerp to Naples and Cologne to Quebec. A church in Rome is dedicated to her as is a shrine in Beaumont-les-Autels, in southern France. On her feast day, dentists from France and nearby countries have traditionally made pilgrimages to this latter site. Her name and spirit were also invoked in the creation of the Guild of St. Apollonia, a charitable dentists group organized in Boston in 1920 to care for the dental needs of the city's parochial-school students. The same city became the home to the Federated Guild of St. Apollonia, another charitable dento-religious organization.

Her imagined likeness has been the subject of many canvases, some by artists of high repute. Originally pictured as an old woman, over time her image became younger and more beautiful. A portrait done in 1670 by Carlo Dolci hangs in the Corsini Gallery in Rome while the Royal Dental Institute of Stockholm has a collection of over 150 different such portraits and pictures, donated by an eminent Stockholm dentist who'd developed more than a professional interest in her. A portrait dating to about 1470 from the school of Piero Della Francesca, now in the collection of the National Gallery of Art in Washington, DC, may look familiar to some. It was the basis for a series of silk screens of St. Apollonia created by Andy Warhol in 1984.

Barberous Operations

MANY REGARD CONTEMPORARY Western civilization as a consumer's paradise, a ceaseless celebration of the service economy in an era of one-stop shopping. A visit to a barber shop can help put this "progress" into perspective. The next time your locks are trimmed, ask the barber or stylist if he or she will extract one of your teeth. Or open a vein and bleed you. Even just perform a minor surgical operation you've been putting off. In all likelihood, your barber will demur. You must go to a different location for each of these services—if you can find anyone to bleed you at all. That's progress.

The Medieval health-care consumer faced no such problem. Long before downsizing and managed care, barber-surgeons brought efficiency to the delivery of a full range of outpatient services.

The St. Peter Principle

BLOODLETTING HAS BEEN used for therapeutic purposes for perhaps 3,000 years. Arising from the humoral school of disease theory, bleeding was used to "regulate" the system. The bleeder's traditional tools were a bowl and staff—not a staff in the sense of the tooth-drawer's motley attendants, but a simple wooden pole. Propped under the patient's arm, the staff helped steady the limb and direct blood into the bowl. This may be the origin of the barber's red-and-white striped pole. The staff may have gotten bloodied as a matter of routine, and possibly been painted red to minimize the garish sight of the blood dripping down the staff. In various illuminated manuscripts, barber-surgeons are identified by a red pole, usually hung at the door, with white bandages wrapped around it.

The union of barbering, bleeding, and surgery extends at least to the early Middle Ages, and their marriage can be said to have been performed at the Vatican. At the time, medicine and surgical operations were performed almost entirely by men in Holy Orders. But the Church hierarchy was increasingly opposed to priests performing any procedure in which blood was shed. Those who did were barred from higher Church offices.

The Papal Decree of 1092 promulgated a new grooming code as well as significant health-care recommendations for monks. It may as well have been drafted by lobbyists for the barber industry. The decree advised turning minor surgery over to barbers (who were accustomed to wielding razors) and directed monks to keep their heads and faces shaved, either to specific styles prescribed for each order or completely bald and beardless. It also called for being bled up to five times a year. For economy's sake, monasteries sought one person who would perform both bleeding and shaving. Soon they were hiring staff barbers. In France they were given the title *rasor et minutor,* or "barber and blood remover." They bled, shaved, and cut hair in the order's signature tonsure, giving rise to their name, *barbi-tonsoribus.* Barbers began performing many surgeries. The skills they learned inside the monastery were applied outside as well.

In 1163, Pope Alexander and the Edict of Tours explicitly banned monks from performing any operation in which blood would be shed. It fell to the barbers who had previously only been their assistants to pick up the scalpel. Tooth extraction was now by papal decree relegated to the realm of nonphysician surgeons, who were considered tradesmen or craftsmen, not health-care professionals. The poorly educated classes included surgeon-barbers, barber-surgeons, and plain barbers.

Monks obviously were not completely following the rules. The Papal Edict of Pope Innocent III in 1215 restated and strengthened the church policy: *Ecclesia abhorret a sanguine*: To shed blood was "incompatible with the divine mission." It was a blanket condemnation on any monk or priest who practiced surgery. "So it fell to barbers, executioners and pig castraters to continue the learning," as one historian noted.

The Guilded Age

REFLECTING THEIR GROWING power, French barbers entered the guilded age with the founding of the Guild of Barbers in Paris in 1210. The word *guild* originally denoted a tax or payment, but came to refer to a trade association or brotherhood of dues-paying members. The barbers' solidarity was soon tested, as a schism erupted in their ranks. Some claimed greater knowledge than others, resulting in a turf war pitting Surgeons of the Long Robe, who considered themselves more surgeons than barbers, against Surgeons of the Short Robe, who were more (or exclusively) barbers than surgeons. Some operations, such as bleeding and the extraction of teeth, were performed by both. As time passed, the groups became more specialized and polarized.

By the 1300s intervention at the highest levels of government was needed to mediate the conflict and regulate their bailiwicks. Royal decrees of the fourteenth century forbade Surgeons of the Short Robe from practicing surgery without first being examined by a Surgeon of the Long Robe. Surgeons of the Short Robe, meanwhile, gradually made procedures including bleeding, leeching, cupping, and the application of enemas their exclusive province.

Across the Channel, English barbers and surgeons were also amalgamating. Barbers of the time "displayed pails of fresh blood, which after congealing were considered less desirable exhibits, and poured to spoil stinking in the streets," according to an account of their promotional practices and disposal methods. The sight and smell of this bloody, stale advertising was unbearable even by London standards. In 1307 the city passed an ordinance stating "no barber shall be so bold or hardy as to put blood in their windows, openly or in view of folks, but let them have it privily carried unto the Thames, under pain of paying two shillings to the use of the sheriffs."

The following year the first known Master of the Barbers, Richard le Barber (or Barbour), was admitted to London's Company of Barbers. The company may have been founded long before that, possibly as a religious organization. The record of Richard's induction, conducted in Latin, notes ". . . And he was admitted and made oath that every month he would make scrutiny throughout the whole of his trade, and if he should find any among them keeping brothels, or acting unseemly in any other way, and to the scandal of the trade, he was to distrain upon them. . . ."

Other companies of the day included grocers, goldsmiths, fishmongers, vintners, skinners, taylors, pewterers, and cutlers.

In 1368 three Master Surgeons were sworn into the company to supervise the practice of surgery. About the same time, a smaller, more select group of surgeons banded together in an unincorporated company, the Fellowship of Surgeons. Of course, these tradesmen could do little to control the practices of noncompany members; others took care of those problems. In 1382 a "counterfeit physician" caught in London "was set on horseback, his face to the horse's tail, the same tail in his hand as a bridle, a collar of Gordans about his neck, a whetstone on his breast and so led through the City of London with ringing of basons, and then banished."

In 1462, Edward IV granted a Royal charter of incorporation to the Company of the Barbers. It omitted from the list of services they were allowed to perform the less respectable activities associated with their trade, such as delousing and brothel-keeping. The charter regulated the practice of surgery, as well. In 1492 King Henry VII granted cognizance to the Fellowship of Surgeons and the following year an informal alliance between the two trade groups was established.

Despite lack of approbation from physicians, the calling of barber and surgeon were obviously important ones. In 1515 Henry VIII ruled that both were, "in consideration of their constant attendance upon patients, exempted by Parliament from all military service."

Henry had already evinced concern with the quality of health-care practitioners in his kingdom. An act passed in 1511 regulating medical and surgical practice and attempting to suppress quacks spelled out why:

Forasmuch as the science and cunning of physick and surgery, is daily within this realm, exercised by a great multitude of ignorant persons, of whom the greater part have no manner of insight in the same, nor any other kind of learning; that common artificers as smiths, weavers and women, boldly and accustomably take upon them great cures and things of great difficulty in which they partly use sorcery and witchcraft, partly apply such medicines unto the disease as to be noxious and nothing more, therefore to the High displeasure of God, great infamy to the Faculty, and the grievous hurt and damage and destruction of many of the King's liege people.

This "ignorant multitude" was hardly the only threat to public health. Throughout the Middle Ages, barber-surgeons, tooth-drawers, and other dental practitioners of the era racked up kill ratios comparable to what a well-equipped and trained combat unit could produce. The toll of their oral ministrations usually landed dentistry firmly in death's top ten list of causes. London's weekly *Bill of Mortality* of August 15–22, 1665, recorded 5,568 fatalities, with "Teeth" holding the no. 5 spot on the chart. Take out the 4,237 dispatched by the plague (the no. 1 killer of the week), and the 111 souls who succumbed to complications from dental procedures accounted for almost 10 percent of all deaths. Most died from "mortification"—infection—that set in after botched operations or as a result of unsanitary practices.

United in Mercantile Matrimony

THE UNION OF barbers and surgeons was formalized in 1540 when a charter from Henry VIII and an Act of Parliament united them, transforming members into "Masters and Governours of the Mystery and Comminalite of Barbours and Surgeons of London." Explicit in this marriage was that tooth-drawing would remain an unregulated field. According to the rules, only company members could practice any "barbery or shavery, surgery, letting of blood, or any other thing belonging to surgery, drawing of teeth only excepted." The charter prohibited surgeons from performing shaves and barbers from practicing surgery—except tooth-drawing.

Rules of conduct for the trade were promulgated—and ignored, as indicated in the pages of the *Annals of the Barber-Surgeons*. The issue of August 26, 1557, noted that Mrs. Dawson, widow of one Bryckette, a tooth-drawer, as per orders, "shall paye no quartryge to the hawse nor hange oute any signe or cloth with teethe as she heretofore hath done." Her offense: after the death of her husband, she remarried, yet carried on his trade, becoming the first woman dentist known to history.

Scurvy had already been taking a toll on English teeth, but the need for dental services of all types increased exponentially as refined sugar became widely available in the seventeenth century. Sugary cakes and marzipan sweetmeats, meat pies topped with a mass of sugar and rosewater, and other sugar-laden foods sent decay rates skyrocketing. Shakespeare's numerous mentions of dental pains and "stinking breath" (dental organs are mentioned in thirty-five of his thirty-seven plays) cannot be attributed to the Bard's well-earned reputation for dramatic invention.

The boom in cavities further fueled the market for magical potions, prayers, and quackery that characterized noninvasive dentistry of the day. Decay respected no class boundaries, save that the commoner was more likely to be spared; they couldn't afford to satisfy their sweet tooth as much as those more financially secure.

Meanwhile, barber-surgeons needed periodic reminders not to leave buckets of blood around for advertising purposes. A 1566 ordinance ordered "that none lett blood stand to the annoyance of the people's," while a 1605 charter simply stated: "No persons to shew his porringers or basons with blood therin."

Eventually buckets of blood lost favor for advertising purposes, replaced by less-perishable but equally attention-grabbing displays. A poem of the early 1700s by John Gay limns the exterior decor of the typical barbers' place of business:

> *His pole with pewter basons hung*
> *Black rotten teeth in order strung,*
> *Rang'd cups, that in the window stood,*
> *Lin'd with red rags to look like blood,*
> *Did well his threefold trade explain,*
> *Who shav'd, drew teeth, and breath'd a vein.*

The Breakup

THE FIRST OBVIOUS signs of marital difficulties between barbers and surgeons came in 1684, when all charters had to be surrendered to the Crown. Concurrently, the surgeons submitted an awkwardly worded petition to Charles II:

> ... it is found by experience that the Union of the Surgeons the person altogether ignorant of the Science or Faculty of Surgery (as the Barbers are) who were heretofore a different Com-

pany from the Surgeons dothe hinder and not promote the order for which they were united, that His Majesty would make that all Surgeons within 7 miles distant thereof a Body Politic under such Regulations as His Majesty shall think fit.

It was a case of incompatibility. As one historian explained, "Physicians thought themselves superior to surgeons, trained surgeons thought themselves above their brethren who also cut hair, while barber-surgeons held ordinary barbers in contempt."

King James II returned the charter unchanged in 1688, but in 1745, by request of the surgeons, parliament split the company into three groups. Elite practitioners united in the Guild of Surgeons. Others formed the Masters and Governors of the Mystery and Commonality of Barbers and Surgeons. The rest banded together in the Master Barbers of London.

Bloodletting remained a regular part of the dental arts. David Perronet, who achieved such success with his universal dentifrice, also highly recommended bloodletting for curing toothaches, and advertised his availability for the procedure:

> I further inform the Public, that I let blood as cheap and safe as any of my profession. I make use of an excellent foreign method of bleeding viz., the observing of the proper times for it. 'Tis common in this country for People to use bleeding, either to prevent sickness, or be cured of some other slight illness, in which case they mind nothing else but their own leisure, or when they can best spare a shilling for it. By the proper time for it, I mean the Moon, which has undoubtedly no small Power over our bodies.

Bloodletting was also practiced by dentists in America, reaching its peak of acceptance in the first half of the 1800s. Before cleaning the teeth or gums, dentists often bled a patient, drawing blood from the arm. It was also recommended as a first step in filling cavities. An article in the debut volume of the *American Journal of Dental Science*, entitled "Of Treating Caries of the Teeth," recommended "local and general bloodletting, etc.," as the standard first step in the treatment of decay.

At the beginning of the twentieth century in England, barbers still performed tooth extractions and bloodletting along with haircutting and shaving.

A Royal Pain

ELIZABETH I WAS continuously afflicted with dental problems in her later years, "a martyr to pyorrhea," as one medical historian wrote after pouring over her records. A German visitor to her court in 1598 reported "her lips are narrow and her teeth black, a defect that the English seem subject to, from their great use of sugar."

By the turn of the century her dental problems had worsened, ultimately costing the queen her front teeth and leading her to adopt cumbersome methods to hide the loss, as described by an intimate in 1602:

> The Queen is still . . . frolicy and merry, only her face showeth some decay, which to conceal when she cometh in public she putteth many fine cloths into her mouth to bear out her cheeks.

Her problematic teeth could make life painful for those around her, as well, as John Strype related in his *Life of Bishop Aylmer,* published in 1701:

> It was in the month of December 1578, when she was so excessively tormented with the Distemper [toothache] that she had no Intermission Day or Night, and it forced her to pass whole Nights without taking any Rest; and came to that Extremity, that her Physicians were called in and consulted. . . . The pulling it out was esteemed by all the safest way; to which, however, the Queen, as was said, was very averse, as afraid of the acute Pain that accompanied it. And now it seems it was that the Bishop of London being present, a Man of high Courage, persuaded her that the pain was not so much, and not at all to be dreaded; and to convince her thereof told her, she should have a sensible Experience of it in himself, though he were an old man, and had not many Teeth to spare; and immediately had the Surgeon come and pull out one of his Teeth, perhaps a decayed one, in her Majestie's Presence. Which ac-

cordingly was done: and She was hereby encouraged to submit
to the Operation herself.

A Mouth with Sex Appeal

EVEN IN THOSE earthier times, a foul mouth was capable of grossing
out members of the opposite sex—especially if one wasn't a king or
queen. *The English Man's Treasure*, published in 1613, offered useful
advice on the subject:

> To take away the stinking of the mouth—wash mouthe with
> water and vinegar and chew masticke then wash mouthe with
> the decoction of Annis seeds, mints and cloves sodden in wine.

Of course there were no toothbrushes for home use—or bathrooms
to hang them in. Barber-surgeons handled teethcleaning, using toothpicks and bits of cloth. After scraping the teeth, they swabbed them
with a stick dipped in *aqua fortis* to whiten them. Strong water, indeed.
It was actually a solution of nitric acid. Although it left the teeth considerably whiter, it achieved this effect by eating away the enamel,
causing the teeth irreparable damage. The ultimate results were bemoaned in *The Jewel House of Art and Nature*, a book which appeared
in 1653:

> And here by those miserable examples that I have seen in some
> of my nearest friends, I am inforced to admonish all men to be
> careful, how they suffer their teeth to be made white with *aqua
> fortis*, which is the Barber's usual water; for unless the same
> be well delayed, and carefully applied, a man with a few dress-
> ings, may be driven to borrow a rank of teeth.

French Class

IN FRANCE, THE more dentally advanced of the two nations, the Faculty
of Medicine of Paris had been giving instructional courses for barber-
surgeons and surgeon-barbers as early as 1505. The lectures were delivered in Latin, the lingua franca of higher education. Thus, they

would have been unintelligible to the vast majority of practicing barbers. The accepted wisdom trumpeted by pedagogues in this moribund
tongue, for example, *lacertae hepat impositum erosis dentibus dolorem
sedat testantur ex aliorum scriptis*, reveals that the impediment to learning posed by the language barrier was probably beneficial. The foregoing gem, for example, can be translated as "lizard liver put into a
carious tooth sedates the toothache, as has been attested in many writings."

Latin had proved invaluable throughout the medieval world for its
ability to obscure the banality and ignorance of what it was employed
to convey. It could also be used in the way parents employ spelling to
encode information in the presence of a young child.

British physician John F. Gaddesden (1280–1361), who taught at
Oxford, demonstrated both the aforementioned principles in a medical
treatise (*Rosa anglica*, printed in 1492) that included the following
instructions for making a painful tooth fall out:

> *Capiatur rana verdis quae de arbore in arborem scandil, et in
> Provincia satis copiose reperitur summatur ipsius adeps et eo
> liniatur dentro quispuis sit et statim excidit.*

To this august advice he added, "Grandeur pecuniam accipi a bar-
bitonsoribus.
Translated into plain English:

> Let a green frog which leaps from tree to tree be seized, and
> in the Province he is found in sufficient abundance, and let his
> fat be taken, and any tooth smeared with it, and immediately
> it falls out.

His aside: "(For this remedy) a great amount of money has been
received from the barbers."

Europe did have its intellectual bright spots amid the Dark Ages.
In Italy, the great medical school at Salerno, civitas Hippocratica, was
formed in 848. Claimed to have been founded by a Greek, a Jew, a
Saracen, and a Latin, this was the site where the world's most famous
medical poem, *Regimen sanitatis salernitatum*, was written over the
course of more then 150 years, perhaps between 1100 and 1250. Running some 3,000 verses in length, it is essentially a "how to" book for

health, offering advice on a variety of ailments. More than 300 editions were printed. At the insistence of Queen Elizabeth, an English version was finally published in 1607. Another English version was printed in Philadelphia in 1870. Dental health was of course addressed. The following verse on treating a toothache is representative of the tome's tenor:

> *If in your teeth you hap to be tormented,*
> *By meane some little wormes therein do breed,*
> *Which paine (if heed be tane) may be prevented,*
> *By keeping cleane your teeth, when as you feed:*
> *Burne Francinsence (a gum not evil sented),*
> *Put Henbane unto this, and Onyon-seed*
> *And with a Tunnel to the tooth that's hollow,*
> *Convey the smoake thereof, and ease shall follow.*
> *By nuts, Oyle, Eeles, and cold in head,*
> *By Apples and raw fruits is hoarsenesse bred.*

3

Is There a *Dentatore* in the House?

Professional Dentistry Emerges in the Glow of the Enlightenment and a Gargle of Urine

T HE YEAR WAS 1527 AND THE FEAST OF ST. JOHN WAS IN FULL swing in Basel, Switzerland. Surely the winds of intellectual freedom blowing across Europe fanned the flames of the roaring bonfire that university students gathered around in celebration that night, a highpoint of the annual revelry. Theophrastus Bombastus Von Hohenheim, now reinvented as Philipus Aureolus Paracelsus, had recently assumed his chair as professor of surgery at the university. He chose this night to inaugurate his lectures, starting with his contribution to the pyre, consigning a copy of Avicenna's *Canon of Medicine,* the day's leading medical textbook, to the flames.

"Into St. John's Fire," Paracelsus announced to the throng, "so that all misery may go into the air with the smoke." His canon shot would echo through the corridors of medical schools from thenceforth. After torching Avicenna, he flamed Galen's writings as well, concluding a celebrity roast that captured the bold spirit of antiauthoritarianism of the day.

An alchemist and physician, Paracelsus (ca. 1493–ca.1541) had taken his adopted name to proclaim his superiority over the famed Roman doctor Celsus. Paracelsus is credited with importing the raw materials of alchemy—sulfur, iron, lead, copper sulfate, arsenic, antimony, and mercury—to the healing arts, thereby introducing chemical pharmacology to Western medicine. The acceptance of his chemically based approach over treatments founded on humoral theories was assisted by contemporary medicine's inability to contain the contagions of the plague and syphilis that ravaged Europe in waves.

Several of the chemicals and elements he introduced would play a large role in the subsequent practice of dentistry and medicine, not infrequently to the detriment of the patient. His most direct dental legacy is said to be the term *tartar*, which he introduced to general medicine, borrowing it from iatrochemist Basil Valentine. He likened the stony accretions to the accumulation of minerals seen in wine casks.

Ultimately Paracelsus was driven out of the city for his unorthodox teaching and intemperate habits. Though he continued to write and teach, he had little further hand in oral research. Historian Hermann Prinz concluded ". . . this man of genius did not contribute anything important to the progress of dentistry," but perhaps Prinz was too harsh in his assessment. Paracelsus is also credited with introducing opium to Western medicine, which would see notable service in dentistry, often relieving the suffering wrought by indiscriminate application of other curative agents he recommended.

Drilling in the Sands of Arabia

CIVILIZATION IN ITS entirety had not been sleepwalking through the Dark Ages. While Europe was locked in its millennium-long funk, the Islamic world grew into a center of progressive intellectualism and inquiry.

The first hint of light preceding Europe's awakening was the landmark writings of Rhazes (ca. 841–926), a Persian physician. His teachings are regarded as the first advances in medical and dental knowledge after the collapse of the Roman Empire, though some hardly seem like forward steps. Rhazes believed toothaches could be caused by heat, inflammation, or cold or thick humors, and each variety was treated differently. For toothaches caused by cold or thick humors, application of theriac (an opium-based medicine), or a mixture of pepper and tar were among the recommended treatments. For "hot" toothaches, he prescribed "cold" substances. Inflamed teeth were treated by cupping or bleeding of veins in the face or temple. Inflamed gums were to be bled, scarified, and cauterized.

Some of Rhazes's recommendations made great sense—like his advice to avoid quacks of all stripes:

> There are so many little arts used by mountebanks and pre-tenders to physic, that an entire treatise would not contain them. Their impudence is equal to their guilt in tormenting persons in their last hours. They profess to cure the falling sickness (epilepsy) by making an issue at the back of the head in the form of a cross. Others give out they can draw snakes out of their patient's noses, or worms from their teeth. No wise man ought to trust his life to their hands.

Avicenna (980–1037), the massively influential physician who authored the *Canon of Medicine* that Paracelsus would later torch, supported both the toothworm and humoral theories of toothache. He recommended fumigation to rid carious teeth of the creatures, as well as shaking sore teeth to expel their morbid humors. He also advocated drilling into these teeth to release the fluids and allow medicine to be directed at the point of distress.

Muslims, like Christian church officials, were averse to spilling blood. Abulcasis (1050–1122), one of the most able writers and surgeons of the medieval world, took a strong interest in dental matters and tried to avoid bloodshed when possible. When he had to perform an extraction, he put sandarach—yellow arsenic sulfide—under the gums a few days before to loosen the tooth. Other Islamic physicians used arsenic to loosen teeth before extraction as well. Syrian remedy of the era called for pouring strong acid on the ground and smearing the resulting seething mud on the bothersome tooth.

Abulcasis was first to write on the treatment of deformities of the mouth and dental arches. A native of Cordova, his monumental *Altasrif* contained a major treatise on surgery divided into three sections. One contained illustrations of dental instruments, the first book in which they are depicted. Fourteen different scrapers and scalers were described, as were the proper way to use them:

> Sometimes on the surface of the teeth, both inside and outside, are deposited rough ugly-looking scales, black, green and yel-low; this corruption is communicated to the gums, and the teeth

are in process of time denuded. Lay the patient's head on your lap and scrape the teeth and molars.

But what he was most concerned about were tonsores—barbers— who practiced surgery in the oral cavity. He advised avoiding all tooth-drawing barbers, ridiculed their techniques and instruments, and complained bitterly that they were permitted to work on teeth— particularly their removal—despite their ignorance.

Abulcasis's complaints are the first known references to barber-surgeons as oral health-care providers. But was his criticism nothing more than professional jealousy? Vincinzo Guerini, the pioneering dental historian, speculates that the tonsores' instruments may have been superior to Albucasis's own.

It is probable . . . that the barbers, in spite of the scorn with which Abulcasis overwhelms them, used, for the extraction of teeth, forceps far more suitable than those described by him. . . . These individuals must have had a great practice in the extraction of teeth . . . as may be argued from the words of Abulcasis himself.

And Abulcasis's extractions were no picnic, despite the sandarach application. He recommended cutting the gums loose, as Celsus had, then gripping the tooth with the fingers and thumb or a pair of pliers and shaking it from side to side. As Guerini noted, "The ignorant barbers, with a speedier method, at least made extraction without pain-killers a less dreadful experience."

Though *fatui tonsores*, silly barbers, as Guerini called them, caused many serious injuries, practitioners of all kinds did the same and worse, as the first death from extraction on record indicates. It was recounted by an Arabian writer, Garriopontus, in 1045:

On the island of Delphi, a painful molar, extracted by (an) inexperienced physician, occasioned the death of a philoso-pher, for the marrow of the tooth, which originates from the brain, ran down the lungs and killed the philosopher.

The exact cause of death is difficult to determine from this description, as is whether the patient would have viewed his impending posthumous honor philosophically.

The thirteenth-century dental gadfly Abd Al-Rahim Al-Jawbari set out to expose the tricks of charlatans and quacks, debunking the toothworm theory and explaining the fraud behind their cures. According to his writings, some embedded a real worm in a cake made from the spurge plant, euphorbia. After the cake was placed in the mouth to soften, the charlatan removed the toothworm using a forceps or his bare fingers. (Chinese charlatans hid maggots in the hollow portion of extricating instruments, and pulled maggots from the mouth along with extracted tooth.)

Al-Jawbari explained the ruse behind fumigation with henbane seeds, as well: Burning the seeds revealed the small embryonic plants inside each seed, which for centuries patients had been told were worms.

A Dental Renaissance

AS THE RENAISSANCE flowered in Italy, dentistry began to blossom. The enriching crosscurrents of arts and science led through the studios of leading artisans as well as medical theorists and practitioners. Benvenuto Cellini (1500–1571), famed Italian sculptor and gold worker, invented a method of casting gold in molds that became the basis for casting gold inlays used in dentistry. Leonardo da Vinci (1452–1519), Mr. Renaissance himself, developed a dramatically advanced description of the anatomy of the teeth and finely detailed renderings of the maxillary sinus.

The convergence of artistry and inquiry was seen in the return and even improvement of dental skills that disappeared with the fall of Rome, such as in the resurrection of fillings. The ancients packed their cavities with all manner of malleable materials, but the advent of metallic fillings came in the late fifteenth century. Giovanni d'Arcoli (ca. 1412–1484), Italian physician and surgeon at Bologna and Padua, wrote of filling teeth with soft, thin gold leaf. From his casual mention of the practice, one can infer this was fairly common at the time, and gold was the metal of choice.

D'Arcoli also developed a unique hypothesis on the cause of tooth-aches that combined the toothworm and humoral theories. Toothworms, he said, arose from spontaneous generation in the morbid humors in the teeth. He also believed some cases resulted from improper digestion, and recommended abstaining from unnecessary movements (including sex and bathing) immediately after meals. Cautery, bloodletting, and laxatives were among the other remedies for toothache he advocated.

In an example of the independent thinking that characterized the times, although most experts advised avoiding tooth-drawers and char-latans, Giovanni d'Vigo (1460–1520), a noted Italian surgeon from Ra-pallo, suggested learning from them:

> For the extraction of teeth there is needed a practical man, and therefore, many medical and surgical authorities expressed an opinion that this operation should be left to expert barbers and to the itinerant quacks who operate in public places. He, therefore, who desires to perform this manual operation in the best manner, will derive great advantage by frequenting men who are experts in performing it, and by seeing and impressing well on his memory their manner of operating.

Vigo wrote learnedly on dental subjects in *Practica in arte chirur-gica*, addressing treatment of dental abscesses and advising on the need for preparing teeth for filling properly. This required careful ex-cavation and shaping of cavities with trephines, files, and scalpels before filling them with gold leaf. To prevent the exposed pulp from infection, some practitioners used arsenic. Though this effectively killed the tissue, the procedure remained in wide use until the intro-duction of Novocain early in the twentieth century.

Patients, not just their teeth, were also being treated in a more enlightened manner. Submitting to treatment had typically been as awkward and humiliating as it was painful. Patients of the era custom-arily lay supine on the floor or ground when receiving dental attention. The operator would get on his knees, and confine the patient's head between them in a grip that has been called viselike. Giocanni Pla-teario (1450–1525), a professor in Pisa, became the first dentist on record to have patients assume a sitting position when undergoing oral ministrations.

Wise Guy

EVER CONCERNED WITH being on the cutting edge, the French were also positioning themselves in the forefront of new dental developments. Guy de Chauliac (1300–1368), most celebrated of the century's surgeons, wrote extensively on dental ailments and operations. His opus, *Chirurgia magna,* was finally printed more than a hundred years after his death (1478) and became a standard text for teaching surgery into the eighteenth century.

A rationalist, de Chauliac helped free medical practice from magic and sorcery as Hippocrates had done over 1,500 years before. A professor at the University of Montpellier, he sympathetically accepted specialists who devoted themselves to the oral cavity, saying "the practice of dental surgery constitutes a specialty," and that "operations on the teeth are appropriate to barbers and *dentatores* to whom the physicians had abandoned them."

He used the term *dentista,* progenitor of the word *dentist,* the first time it is found in print. He also used the terms *dentateur* and *dentator.*

A proponent of the worm theory of tooth decay, he suggested fumigation with seeds of leek, onion, and henbane mixed with goat's tallow to drive out the worms. Bloodletting from the lips, tongue, and facial veins were other treatments he advocated. For pain management during operations, de Chauliac recommended knocking out patients using decoctions of opium, hyoscyamine, and lettuce.

Advances in nondental medicine found their way mouthward as medical pioneers dabbled in oral research. France's Ambroise Paré (1510–1590), owner of the honorific, "Father of Modern Surgery," has been said to also qualify for the title, "Foster Father of Dental Surgery."

He began his career in a barber shop. Naturally, the position required surgical skills, and his natural abilities in this arena were soon noted. In short order he was under the command of the armed forces, working as a military surgeon. The fearsome wounds produced by canon, firearms, and other state-of-the-art weapons gave him an extensive education in prosthetic appliances as well as surgical skills. At the time, wounds were treated with boiling oil and by searing the flesh. Paré threw out his searing tools and gave his brazier and oil pots to his cook, treating the wounded with only soothing emollients and bandages. The increase in survival rates was dramatic, earning Paré the animosity of his colleagues.

Returning to civilian life, he brought reform to surgical education and practice, and championed the same principles in dentistry:

> The extraction of a tooth should not be carried out with too much violence, as one risks producing luxation of the jaw or concussion of the brain and the eyes, or even bringing away a portion of the jaw together with the tooth (the author himself has observed this in several cases), not to speak of other serious accidents which may supervene, as, for example, fever, apostema, abundant hemorrhage, and even death.

Yet Paré seemed to bring the standard "take no prisoners" attitude to the extractions he occasionally performed, judging from accounts of his standard operating procedure. First he used a *dechaussoir* to loosen gum tissue from tooth, then a *poussoir* to push the tooth from the socket, and for the coup de grâce, the *davier*, or pelican, to lift it from the alveolus, or tooth socket.

His claim to paternity of dental surgery is based in part on his pioneering work with dental prostheses, having made the first prosthetic plate for cleft palates.

Most physicians of Paré's day retained their long-standing repugnance for both dentistry and surgery. If a physician sought to remove a tooth, it would be done *sine ferro*, or without iron, as opposed to *cum ferro*. Tinctures—actually strong acids—were often used over a period of time to loosen teeth prior to extraction. Meanwhile, the Church remained a major impediment to progress. The wisdom of the ancients was held unassailable. Religious dogma demanded faith in both God and Aristotle.

Andreas Vesalius (1514–1564), the Father of Anatomy, challenged accepted knowledge of the day, contradicting Galen's theories and fostering interest in anatomy. His student, Gabriele Fallopio, devoted most of his attention not to dental caries, but to cavities of a different sort. He coined the terms *vagina* and *clitoris*, and detailed the eponymous fallopian tubes in his only published work, *Observationes anatomicae*, published in 1561. He also investigated the oral cavity, and described the development of the teeth in great detail, becoming the first author to describe the dental follicle.

Church opposition to dissection had long made research in these areas problematic. Cadavers were not legally available for slicing and dicing. The unquenchable demand for research subjects led to the morgue and graveyard. A thriving market in "bootleg" bodies, uprooted from their recent resting place or stolen before they ever hit the ground, developed even before the Renaissance. A signal event in the trade was the first criminal prosecution for body snatching in 1319.

The Golden Tooth

WHILE DENTISTRY MARCHED forward, ignorance had not been standing motionless. The field remained fertile for fraud, quackery, and bunkum, often promulgated or promoted by the learned of the day. Few examples are more instructive than the late sixteenth-century case known as the Story of the Golden Tooth. It first came to widespread attention with the publication of Professor Jacob Horst's *De auro dente maxillari puer Silesii* in 1593. The professor, on the medical faculty at Germany's University of Helmstedt, reported on a seven-year-old Silesian boy from whose gums a golden tooth had erupted. The precious metal molar, first on the left side of the lower jaw, had been examined by many experts and adjudged a surprisingly highly refined grade, on a par with coin gold. Many pamphlets were published about this marvel, probing its provenance in the most learned terms.

Horst concluded that the golden tooth was created by a supernatural power as a result of the peculiar planetary alignment under which the youth was born. On his birth day, the sun was in the sign of the ram in conjunction with saturn, producing intense heat that caused gold matter, rather than tooth substance, to be secreted when the tooth formed. He likened the tooth to an earthquake, eclipse, or comet, a portent of momentous events to come, in this case the destruction of the enemies of Christianity by the Roman emperor.

Research was hampered by the youngster's reticence to open his mouth. The boy's stubbornness provoked a nobleman to stab his face with a dagger, wounding him severely enough to require surgery. While the repairs were being effected, the mystery of the tooth's origin became clear. One of the cusps of the molar had begun to penetrate through the gold cap, revealing the Golden Tooth for the hoax it was: a well-fitting gold shell crown. Yet the fraud indicates someone at the time was proficient with the merging of metal and mouth, a combination that would prove so important to the practice of dentistry. The boy, meanwhile, was packed off to prison.

A somewhat similar account appeared in Poland in 1674 by a Jesuit father in Vilna. *Disquisitio physica,* described another unusual first molar, this one in the mouth of a three-year-old. But rather than a golden color, this one appeared more yellowish. The explanation for this, it was determined, was a massive buildup of tartar.

Such was the climate that nurtured the growth of inquiry during the Enlightenment. By the time Paracelsus ignited his students passion with his fiery act of intellectual insubordination, the winds of change had risen to gale force. The Church could no longer control its violent drafts.

Reading the Fine Print—The Beginning of Dental Literature

WITH THE INVENTION of the movable-type printing press by Johannes Gutenberg (ca. 1390–1468) in 1450, dentistry could establish a literary tradition in earnest. The ensuing onslaught of books and pamphlets cemented dentistry's identity as an independent medical specialty. It also allowed misconceptions and fallacies preserved on parchment and spread orally to enjoy wider dissemination.

In 1530, the first book devoted entirely to dentistry, the anonymously published *Zene Artzney,* or "Medicines for the Teeth" (also printed as *Artzney Buchlein*) appeared in Germany. A small booklet, its forty-four pages discussed topics including loose teeth, decay, and toothworms. Written in German, rather than Latin, it found an enthusiastic readership, and was widely used by uneducated barbers, barber-surgeons, and surgeons as a training manual.

"What toothache or pains in the teeth are, know no one better than he who has experienced them, and I think there are no greater pains than these," the author wrote, suggesting a variety of treatments. But, "If the pains cannot be quieted in any way, in order not to produce damage to the other teeth or pains, you must take refuge in the last resort, i.e., to draw out the bad teeth, which must be done by a person experienced in these things, as drawing out injudiciously is liable to do damage." After describing the correct procedure, the book offered hints on how to tell if any collateral damage had occurred.

The sign by which you may judge whether the jaw be fractured or something of it broken off, is when the cavity wherefrom the tooth has been drawn bleeds more than usual, and the jaw swells so much that one cannot open the mouth, and the cavity festers and swells.

By the time the last version was published in 1576, it had been through fourteen editions.

Reflecting a hegemony in publishing rather than dentistry, the second important work on this field, *Useful Instructions on the Way to Keep Healthy, to Strengthen and Reinvigorate the Eyes and Sight with Further Instructions on the Way of Keeping the Mouth Fresh, the Teeth Clean, and the Gums Firm,* was also produced in Germany. Written by by Walter Hermann Ryff in about 1544, it explained, in part, the close connection between the subjects of its title.

The eyes and the teeth have an extraordinary affinity or reciprocal relation to one another, by which they very easily communicate to each other their defects and diseases, so that they one cannot be perfectly healthy without the other being so too.

Ryff's subsequent works, *Minor Surgery* and *Major Surgery,* included illustrations of many contemporary dental instruments. His detailed drawings of forceps, pelicans, elevators, sealers, tongue scrapers, and excavators are enough to make one wince. Yet an illustration of the wiring of a broken mandible, along with the requisite instruments for its repair, speaks to the evolving sophistication of oral care.

It was also during this era that Hieronymus Cardanus (1501–1576) noted that some teeth erupted later than others, and that due to the delayed appearance of the third molars, they were called wisdom teeth.

A voice of reason was heard from Spain in 1557, with the publication of a slight book by physician Francisco Martinez, containing a conversation about the worm theory of decay. A character named Valerio avows: "I say there are no worms involved in tooth decay, but rather that it is simply corruption, and that the fumigation with henbane constitutes their origin and is a fraud."

Another widely noted early work was Johann Stephan Strobelberger's *De dentium podagra,* loosely translated as "The tooth's Footache" or "Gout in the Teeth." Published in 1630, it compiled dental remedies and treatments of the era, most of them questionable. Strobelberger was the physician at the Royal Baths of Carlsbad. He probably did not perform services offered by barber-surgeon attendants at the less prestigious bath houses of the lower classes. Thus, he himself may have never pulled a tooth, applied a leech or a cup, or perhaps even lanced a boil. In place of instruments for extraction, Strobelberger recommended the fat of a green tree frog. Given the ubiquity of this advice in books on dentistry, one must assume such creatures were exceedingly difficult to catch or nonexistent.

Some historians proclaim Strobelberger's work a clear retrogression in dental literature when compared with *Zene Artzney*. Yet Guerini finds significance in the work: "It gives us a clear idea of the pitiful state in which the dental art still was in the first half of the seventeenth century."

All these and other books and pamphlets that appeared during the first three decades of dental literature were aimed at the mainstream market. The first book on dentistry for a professional audience, *Libellus de dentibus*, by Bartolommeo Eustachio, rolled off the press in Venice in 1563. The first complete volume on the anatomy of the teeth, it included detailed descriptions of their embryology and physiology.

The dental book proved a publishing success story. By the end of the sixteenth century, more than forty books on dentistry and dental anatomy had been published on the continent. But while Europe was awash in dental tomes, the English showed as little regard for dental books as many of them did for the appearance of their teeth. The first book on dentistry in English wasn't printed until about 1687, with the publication of Charles Allen's *Curious Observations in that Difficult Part of Chiururgery Relating to the Teeth, Showing How to Preserve the Teeth and Gums from All Accidents They Are Subject To*. Even if the fifty-six-page booklet broke little new ground, at least it broke the language barrier.

Dawn of the Dentist

WHILE CHARLATANS HELD sway on the Pont-Neuf, Paris was gaining a reputation as the continent's capital of dental excellence. University-trained dental specialists dubbed *dentateurs* had been plying their trade since the early 1500s. They were granted a variety of appellations to distinguish them from barbers and teeth surgeons. Grads hung up shingles as *operateur pour le mal des dents* (operators for tooth ailments), *expert pour les dents* (dental expert), and *Chirgurgien-operateur* (surgeon operator).

By 1622 some French practitioners were operating with the title of surgeon-dentist. Credit for advances of the era could be claimed in no small part by Louis XIV (1638–1715), the Sun King. The lavish seasonal encampment at Versailles, highpoint of social circuit of the era's Eurotrash, placed a premium on appearance, youthfulness, physical beauty, and bodily perfection. Teeth were a critical part of the package. The resulting demand for restorative work and dentures created a supply of advanced dental craftsmen.

By the end of the 1600s even English tooth-drawers were making advances in their trade. Perhaps seeking to escape their past, they took to calling themselves "operators for the teeth," while continuing to specialize in extractions.

Views of the teeth and mouth changed forever in 1683 when Anton van Leeuwenhoek of Delft, Holland, turned his newly invented microscope on scrapings from the teeth. His discovery, a teeming, overwhelming population of *animacules,* left him groping for comparison: "The number of these animals in the scurf of a man's teeth are so many that I believe they exceed the number of men in the Kingdom."

The eighteenth century brought the true birth of dentistry, and wasted no time ushering in the new era. In 1700, the French College of Surgeons opened a department of *Chirurgiens Dentistes*—dental surgeons. Following this date, graduates were compelled to submit to regular examinations, and as one historian notes, "from this period we must date, in modern times, the regular establishment of this art as a distinct branch of surgical practice."

That same year in London, anatomist William Cowper (1666–1709) boldly moved dentistry into the antrum, or sinus cavity, when he performed the first known extraction of a permanent molar involving the maxillary sinus. Probably the first surgeon to treat a diseased antrum, the technique he used to gain access, described in print by a contemporary, James Drake, is still known to dental surgeons as the Cowper-Drake operation.

It must have been a bracing climate for a prospective young dentist—a youngster like Pierre Fauchard (1678–1761)—to grow up in.

Known today by his honorific, "the Father of Dentistry," he would leave extra-large footprints on the pages of oral history.

The Father of Dentistry

PIERRE FAUCHARD'S 1728 opus, *Le Chirurgien Dentiste* and its two subsequent editions (1756 and 1786), is considered a landmark in oral care, it's publication signaling the beginning of the modern era of dentistry.

Fauchard railed against the quackery of the day, even as he offered questionable cures of his own: Gargling with urine to cure a toothache, for example. "One should retain it some time in the mouth and continue its use," he advised.

Born in Brittany about 1678, the games and play of childhood held little interest for young Pierre, and "never distracted me from surgery to which I was destined from my youth," he later wrote. He received his initial dental training in the King's Navy, a subject in which all naval surgeons were schooled. With scurvy, misfiring canons, drunken fist fights, and other oral hazards of the seafaring life, surely he was exposed to a variety of challenging cases. He had the benefit of an excellent teacher in surgeon major M. Alexandre Poteleret, an expert in diseases of the mouth. "I owe him the first glimmerings of knowledge which I acquired in surgery, which I practice, and the progress which I made with this able man has stimulated me later on to make considerable discoveries," he wrote.

Following his naval service, Fauchard went into private practice in Paris and became one of the city's top dentists. Awareness of the tooth's oftimes cruel dichotomy informed all his writing: "The teeth in the natural condition are the most polished and the hardest of all the bones of the human body; but at the same time they are the most subject to diseases which cause acute pain, and sometimes become very dangerous," he noted, a "sad experience" that "we all have."

Yet what happened after the pain began could be even sadder, he warned. "Nothing is more common than for a person to go to the nearest place to have a tooth drawn, it is with difficulty that they are made to understand the danger to which they are sometimes exposed by an operation which appears so simple and so common."

He showed tremendous skill in his prosthetic work and great dexterity and ingenuity with ligatures. These were the silk, linen, and metal threads used to fasten artificial teeth and bridges in place by attaching them to neighboring teeth. He pioneered fastening principles that hold crown and bridgework in place today, relying on roots for the support of artificial crowns and removing pulp remnants from diseased teeth.

A keen observer and bold thinker, Fauchard revolutionized dentistry in part simply by promulgating all he knew. Previous practitioners had done their best to conceal whatever wisdom they thought they possessed. Fauchard gathered his knowledge in the monumental *The Surgeon Dentist.* Its raison d'être was spelled out in the subtitle:

Or A Treatise on the Teeth in which is seen the means used to keep them clean and healthy, of beautifying them, of repairing their loss and remedies for their diseases and those of the gums and for accidents which may befall the other parts in their vicinity with observations and reflections on several special cases.

Dentistry du Jour

THE SURGEON DENTIST reveals not only its author's perspicacity, but also dentistry as practiced by many of his contemporaries and its toll on patients. The problem with dentistry, as Fauchard saw it, was the surgeons. "The most famous surgeons having abandoned this part of the art, or at least having paid little attention to it, have caused by this negligence, the rise of people who without theory or experience, have degraded it, and practiced haphazard, without principles or method."

Take the case of M. Henri Amariton, who "was greatly incommoded by the size and position of a canine" in about 1730. The unhappy results were recorded in a chapter, "On a tooth forced into the maxillary sinus on the right by a charlatan, and on the consequences of this accident."

Amariton's first molar on the right side of his upper jaw hurt, and given "the discomfort and pain which this tooth caused to the gentleman decided him to have it drawn." Amariton made the decision to give up his tooth at the beginning of Lent, though Fauchard is silent on any religious connection. The extraction was handled by a practitioner identified as la Roche Operator, residing in Nonette. Placing his patient in "what he thought was the most suitable position," Mssr. Operator gripped the tooth with a dental key, picked up a stone, and began hammering on the key. The blows drove the tooth "almost obliquely across the maxillary sinus so that it was no longer visible."

"When the tooth had thus disappeared, this empiric assured those present that the patient had swallowed it. This appeared quite probable since they had searched for the tooth without being able to find it."

Amariton sought medical attention for his continuing discomfort, but physicians were unable to ascertain the cause of the "little hard tumor without inflammation" which appeared on the patient's cheek near the nose. Several consultations with surgeons in the town of Clermont failed to find the cause. It was only after he consulted Parisian surgeons that the problem was identified. The tooth had to be extricated by "cutting through the gums, seizing the roots with straight pincers, and yanking out the whole tooth."

Fauchard attributed the high accident rates from dental procedures in part to the variety of unqualified people from unrelated professions offering oral health-care services. He professed that

> So many meddle in work on the teeth although they are of another profession, that I think that presently there will be more dentists than people with toothaches. There are indeed certain cutlers who meddle with extraction of the teeth. Apparently the instruments which they make gives them an itch to try them. I have known one in this town who passes in his quarter as a tooth-drawer. This particular man who had seen several charlatans operate, thinking that it would be as easy to draw teeth as to make knives, has joined the ranks and does not defer when the opportunity offers to put his pretended skill into practice, and his instruments of the proof; and if he does not always take out the tooth whole he does manage to take a piece of it.

He related the case of another cutler, whom he termed a "famous operator," who was called on to examine a youngster whose molar was pitted with black spots. He decided it had to be pulled.

He attempted to draw it, but having only removed the crown (because it was only a milk tooth which was ready to fall out) this new doctor whose discernment was too limited to be able to judge, thought he had made a mistake and had broken the tooth. In order not to leave the operation without completing it he drew also the pretended root of this tooth, when he was astonished to see that it was an entire tooth and not a root, and that it was precisely what which as to have replaced the crown of the first tooth he had drawn. . . . This cutler had however sufficient presence of mind not to acquaint those present at this fine operation, and sent this young person away less rich by one tooth of which the loss will be always a testimony to the ignorance and the temerity of this worthy operator, and to the imprudence of confiding indifferently to these people.

Tools of the Trade

FOR HIS OWN extractions, Fauchard described five kinds of instruments for drawing teeth he used, available to all dentists: the gum lancet, the punch, the pincers, the lever, and the pelican. The gum lancet detached the gums from the body of a tooth or roots. The punch to push a tooth or stump inward in its sockets for removal. Pincers pinched the body of the tooth to help remove it. The lever, or elevator, designed to lift the tooth, was more likely to break the tooth than to draw it out, he said. His primary extraction tool was the pelican.

The pelican was said to be named for its inward pointing hooks, which resembled the beak of the aqueous avian. A religious derivation of the name has also been suggested, as one of Christ's honorifics in the Middle Ages was the Pelican of Grace. Surely anyone facing its use could feel abandoned by God.

Fauchard also described a new kind of pelican capable of pulling teeth "which cannot be drawn as easily with any other instrument." Yet the implement was also capable of unmatched dental destruction.

Of all the instruments used for drawing the teeth, a pelican, such as the one I have described, appears to me the most useful. It's effect is more prompt, more sure than that of any of the others when one knows how to handle it, without which the pelican, however, perfect it may be, is the most dangerous of all instruments for drawing teeth.

Despite his preoccupation with dentistry, Fauchard viewed the mouth holistically. That, along with standard remedies of the day, are documented in one of the cases described in *Four Observations on Violent Pains in the Head Caused by the Teeth*. The patient was Madame de Maubreuil, a Nantes resident affected with headaches in 1715. She had already exhausted the abilities of her physician and surgeon by the time she came to Fauchard.

"This lady was bled and purged several times but as her trouble did not lessen, these gentlemen ordered baths and the application of leeches to her head. She fulfilled their commands to the letter. None of these remedies gave her any relieve whatever," Fauchard reported.

This lady had two decayed teeth which for a long time had given pain and interfered with eating. That made me think that they might be the cause of all the ills from which she suffered. As I had the honor of being well known to her, she resolved to seek me at Angers where I lived at that time. When she came to me I examined her mouth, and found that she had two very carious molars one on the right side of the lower jaw and the other on the left. I considered that these two teeth were alone the cause of her headache and I determined then to extract them which I had no sooner done than this lady found that she was entirely relieved of a pain which had tormented her for six months."

In 1729, Fauchard became the first dentist known to place patients in a chair, instead of having them sit on the floor as was customary. He recommended using a conventional armchair for the purpose. Not all his recommendations were as easy to follow. The mouthwashes, mixtures, and opiates he advised rinsing with could be difficult to create, as a single concoction could call for ingredients as diverse as a couple of ounces of prepared coral, an ounce of dragon's blood, some cachou and gambia along with cinnamon, cloves, and poisonous pyrethrum (chrysanthemum) root, today used in insecticides. Cuttlefish bone as well as burnt eggshells could be required, and the whole pulverized potion might have to be passed through a silk sieve before it could be mixed "with sufficient honey of roses" to allow its use.

He was not immune to the day's fallacies, either. He advocated bloodletting for relief of toothaches. And though not a toothworm proponent per se, he left open the possibility that insect larvae hatched in the mouth could cause itching and dull pain. However, toothworms were coming closer to eradication in the minds of rational practitioners. In 1757 an evangelical pastor, Jacob Christian Schaffer, published an exposé, *The Fancied Worms in Teeth,* debunking the toothworm theory, adding one more voice to the parade of luminaries who had renounced the creatures as frauds. Yet, these hearty creatures would remain alive in some cultures into the twentieth century.

Dentists Cross the Channel

IN THE MID-1600s, a few English practitioners began referring to themselves as "operators for the teeth," Anglicizing the job title popularized by the French. This new breed typically began their careers as apprentices to barbers, scraping and pulling teeth, or working with ivory or smithing gold. Peter de la Roche is credited by some with being London's first, and was by appointment "Operator to the King's teeth." Another of his patients was the wife of diarist Samuel Pepys. The tribulations of her poor dentition are recorded in Pepys' diary, though every so often there was a good news to record, as on the evening of march 11, 1661: "At night home and found my wife come home, and she had got her teeth new done by la Roche, and are indeed now pretty and handsome, and I was much pleased with it."

Tools of the extraction trade in the eighteenth century remained virtually indistinguishable from torture devices. Bleeding, dosing, and enemas remained the cornerstones of medicine. Instruments for cleaning teeth included the euphonious graver, chisel, knife, and z-shaped hook.

A new innovation in extraction tools was introduced early in the century: the dental key, or simply, key. Origin unknown, the first detailed description appeared in 1725. It looked like a hybrid created by sticking the moveable head of a pelican to the end of an old-fashioned door key, like a corkscrew with a gripping claw instead of a pointy twist at the end. By the 1770s the key was the extraction instrument of choice among dentists. It was designed to work fast, an imperative for extraction devices in preanesthetic times. After hooking the claw over the crown, a brisk turn on the handle was supposed to be sufficient to break the tooth from its socket. The popularity of the device can be surmised from its common nomenclature. The English called it the German key and the Germans called it *Clavis Anglica,* or the English key. The French referred to it as the English Key, as well as *le clef de Frere Come,* in honor of a cleric who supposedly improved the design.

Given the horror these tools provoked, powders and tinctures promising immunity from dental problems remained hugely popular. The advertisement for one such powder, hawked in the *Daily Courant* in 1717 is typical:

> It at once makes the teeth as white as ivory, tho' never so black or yellow, and effectually preserves them from rotting or decaying, continuing them sound to exceeding old age. It wonderfully cures the scurvy in the gums, prevents rheum or defluxions, kills worms at the root of the teeth, and thereby hinders the tooth-ache. It admirably fastens loose teeth, being a neat and cleanly medicine of a pleasant and graceful scent.

In the late 1750s the word *dentist* entered the English language. It was adapted, as so many were, from the French word, *dentiste.* Tooth-drawers also continued using a variety of other names borrowed from the French, like "operator for the teeth," and "surgeon operator." The plethora of names was remarked on in the *London Chronicle* in April of 1764:

> Every tooth-drawer who pretends to draw with a touch, is an Operator for the Teeth at least; the renowned Chevalier is indeed only Imperial, Royal, and Pontificial Opthalmiater in the whole world; Mr. Paul Jullion the only Rectifier of Deficient Heads; but Occulists and Dentists abound in every country town; and I cannot help smiling at the rustic Barber Surgeon, who joined both together and stile himself on his shop-board, *Occulis for the Teeth.*

Unlike tooth-drawers, however, those who called themselves dentists didn't perform extractions initially. Instead they offered a range of other dental services and treatments. Like their predecessors, though, they were largely self-taught, and would remain that way for more than a century. An 1840s observer noted that to practice dentistry, "a brass plate and brazen effrontery (were) all the diplomas necessary."

A smattering of knowledge of treatment was beneficial, of course. Aspiring dentists garnered tips from advertising leaflets circulated by equally unqualified rivals. Prospective practitioners also became acolytes of established dentists—some of whom proved surprisingly adept and brought honor and credit to the nascent field. Trainees might sign up for a short course of a few weeks time or become a full-fledged apprentice devoting four or five years of their young lives learning the craft. One English trainee of the era described his education:

The mode of instructing me that Mr. Sheffield adopted was to work with me at the bench and occasionally to take me into his surgery, where I saw him operate. I was also at his side when he saw the gratis patients who came to him each morning at nine o'clock to be relieved of pain. I did all his mechanical work during my apprenticeship, and after about three months he gave the care of the gratis patients into my hands, and I well remember when I went down alone to extract my first tooth, which I am happy to say I accomplished successfully.

The first important book written in English on dentistry appeared during this time, as well, Thomas Berdmore's *Disorders of Deformities of the Teeth and Gums* (1768). Berdmore, dentist to King George III, suggested using microscopes to examine structure of the teeth, discussed the role of sugar in tooth decay, and revealed the results of his studies on the abrasive properties of the tooth powders of the day. His research proved the dentifrices were effective at removing stains from the teeth—and much more. He found brushing a tooth for about an hour with some powders was sufficient to wear away the tooth's enamel.

Without brushing, however, almost the opposite could happen, owing to rapid accumulation of tartar, as observed in one case he recounted:

A gentleman of the Bank, not above twenty-three years of age, applied to me for advice concerning his Teeth . . . which gave him constant pain. I found them perfectly buried in Tartar, by which each set was united in one continuous piece, without any distinction, to show the interstices of the teeth, or their figure or size. The stony crust projected a great way over the gums on the inner side, as well as on the outer, and pressed upon them so hard as to have given rise to the pain he complained of. Its thickness at the upper surface was not less than half an inch . . .

His most famous patient, the king, was not above his subjects when it came to suffering toothaches. At the conclusion of one such episode, the king was about to have a tooth extracted, and confessing fear, called for a glass of brandy before the operation. Though it is not noted whether Berdmore was the dentist in attendance, when the wine was brought, the king had the dentist present it to him. King George III declined to take the glass, saying, "I have no need of it; but was merely anxious to observe if your hand was steady."

An English Transplant

LONG IN THE shadows of French dental pioneers, England finally produced a homegrown oral visionary in the person of John Hunter (1728–1793). His *Natural History of the Human Teeth, Explaining Their Structure, Use, Formation, Growth and Diseases,* published in 1771, formed the foundation for modern anatomical texts on the teeth and jaws. With its supplement, *A Practical Treatise on the Diseases of the Teeth,* published in 1778, Hunter ushered in the era of scientific dentistry.

Hunter had distinguished himself as a surgeon before turning his attention to the teeth. His recommended treatments have been called "signally extraordinary." Certainly they are unusual by today's standards. For affected molars he recommended extraction, followed by immediate boiling and replacement of the tooth in the alveolar socket. Having been rendered "dead" by the boiling, he claimed, the tooth was now immune from further disease. Patients who opted to forego this protocol faced Hunter's backup therapy: burning the nerve of the affected tooth with concentrated sulfuric acid, nitric acid, or other toxic chemical. If the pain was restricted to the tooth, he advised a remedy more aural than oral: burn the ear with hot irons.

Hunter, displaying an aversion to book learning from a young age, had only a rudimentary education. Since he wasn't a dentist, he had no practical experience effecting the treatments he recommended. This "lack of intimate knowledge" of the subject, as one historian called it, led some subsequent writers to condemn him for shortsightedness, lack of qualifications, and discouragement of dental research. Such concerns had no impact on the acceptance of his work at the time or its standing today.

As wrong as he was about some dental matters, he showed a surprising prescience in others. His writings on *Extraneous Matter upon the Teeth*, what we call plaque today, can be seen as a seminal document in the field of oral hygiene. He stated that eating fruits and salads would prevent the buildup of what we know as salivary calculus, through the action of their acids on "preventing the formation of deposits."

Hunter was also celebrated for a feat that would have been branded magic a century before, but could now be explained by science: successfully transplanting a budding human tooth germ into a rooster's comb, where it firmly rooted. The success fired his drive to try similar methods in humans, leading to a tooth transplantations craze.

Human tooth transplants had been mentioned by Paré in 1564 and referred to disparagingly by Charles Allen in his book in 1685. But Hunter's experiments and writing created a rage for them. He used freshly harvested teeth, and advised keeping several potential donors close at hand to assure a wide selection in filling a customer's empty socket. If the first donor's tooth failed to fit the socket correctly—after it had been yanked—on to the second. Once implanted, the new tooth was tied to neighboring teeth until the transplant stabilized.

Advertisements for natural human teeth donors were frequently placed in leading daily papers from 1750 to about 1840 in both England and America. One placed in New York's *Independent Journal* in 1783 is typical:

Any person disposed to part with their front teeth may receive Two guineas for each Tooth, on applying at No. 28 Maiden Lane.

The procedure was rarely successful for more than a few months, yet tooth transplantation would remain popular in England and parts of America until early in the nineteenth century. And successful or not, they were being performed by dentists, now a recognized, if not always respected, class of practitioners.

Hanky-Panky

ETIQUETTE INVOLVING THE teeth and their care was also evolving. On the continent, an empress's bad teeth rehabilitated a disgraced fashion accessory. The empress was Josephine and the item was the handkerchief, which had acquired a certain shock value in France, something not fit to be displayed in proper company. Josephine felt her teeth were even less fit to be seen, she may have been correct judging from remarks of contemporaries. One female acquaintance cattily commented, "Her very small mouth artfully concealed her bad teeth."

The empress was said to have spent hours in front of a mirror learning to smile without showing her teeth. But this simple artifice wasn't enough, so she turned for concealment to an article sure to have a similar shock value as her teeth: the hankie.

"She was in the habit of carrying small handkerchiefs, which she constantly raised gracefully to her lips," according to one account. Said one bureaucrat after meeting her, "she laughed until she cried—never forgetting, however, to put her hankie to her lips to conceal her dreadful teeth."

Ladies of the court followed her example, and handkerchiefs soon became a fixture of the "feminine toilet" of the era, turning the disgraced snot rag into a de rigeur fashion accessory.

Much less concerned with appearances or propriety was Prince von Kaunitz-Rietberg (1711–1794), a prominent Austrian statesman. His habits were described as "especially revolting" by dental historian Gardner Foley. Countess Potockai gave an account of them in her memoirs:

As soon as the table was cleared his valet put a mirror, a basin and brushes before him, and then and there the prince began his morning toilet over again, just as if he had been alone in his dressing room, while every one was waiting for him to finish to get up from the table.

After dinner the prince treated us with the cleaning of his gums, one of the most nauseous operations I have ever witnessed, and it lasted a prodigiously long time, accompanied with all manner of noises. He carries a hundred implements in his pockets for this purpose—glasses of all sorts for seeing before and behind his teeth, a whetting steel for his knife, pincers, and knives and scissors without number."

4

The American Experience

Dental Care Comes to the New World,
Sparking a Revolution

T HE WIDE-OPEN SPACES OF THE NEW WORLD INSPIRED A practical-minded ingenuity and revolutionary zeal in early American dentistry. Yet New World dental history was being written—or drilled and filled—long before our forepatients arrived from the Old World.

Indigenous Dentition

NATIVE DIETS OF simple grains, fruits, and vegetables deprived indigenous populations of naturally occurring cavitation, so they created their own. The rich record of teeth mutilation practiced in Central and South America attests to their skill in this regard. A popular cosmetic operation among pre-Columbian societies, many skulls have been found sporting teeth decorated with inlays of gold, jadeite, hematite, turquoise, rock crystal, or obsidian. Primitive bow drills are thought to have been used to create the man-made cavities in which the precious minerals and metals were set. Circular disks of gold, for example, were inserted into the front of upper incisors, giving owners a rich, dotted smile. Dental remains also reveal a fondness for filing teeth in so called "Sun God fashion," named for a Mesoamerican solar deity traditionally depicted with similarly filed teeth.

North American tribes didn't exhibit the same sophistication in their toothwork, but like their cousins to the south, decay was rare.

They attributed their excellent dental health to the use of tobacco and magic. Toothaches were not unknown, though, and several therapies were available. Among them: cut out a piece of sod before sunrise, breathe upon it three times, and restore it to the place it was taken from. Preventive dentistry was addressed, as well. To avoid losing a tooth, one was advised to spit upon seeing a shooting star. To insure a tooth would stay sound throughout life, catch a green snake, stretch it horizontally by the neck and tail, move it seven times back and forth, then turn it loose. Afterward, eat no food prepared with salt for four days.

In the mid-1800s, Rev. William Leach of Omaha, Nebraska, described a Pawnee medicine man's treatment that was probably similar to what had been practiced for centuries. The medicine man had been summoned to treat an inflamed third molar of one Running Wolf. The healer, according to Leach, "danced around the patient in a semicircle, rattling a gourd . . . [then] he took a small stone knife and cut an 'x' on Running Wolf's cheek, directly over the throbbing tooth. He sucked at the cut lightly . . . [and] pretended to draw out the fang . . . then dashed it into the fire. 'The Evil Spirits cannot use it again,' he said triumphantly." The patient, according to Leach, was thus fooled into believing his tooth had been removed.

A rapid decline in Native American oral health was seen following the arrival of European settlers, due to the introduction of Old World cuisine.

A Deadly Dental Problem

ALTHOUGH AMERICAN DENTISTRY can't claim to have arrived on the *Mayflower*, an extracting tool combining a lever, elevator, and forceps did, as part of the ship's surgical case. Dentistry landed in the New World a decade later, on July 6, 1630, with a fleet of fourteen ships and 1,500 immigrants. Boston was the port of call. Three barber-surgeons, dispatched by the Council for New England (an enterprise formed in the wake of the reorganization of its parent corporation, the Plymouth Company), were among the arrivistes. One can scarcely imagine their thoughts and fears as they contemplated this brave New World, given the low pool of potential patients and high degree of competition. One barber-surgeon, William Dinly, encountered the very problem that had driven many colonists out of England in the first instance: religious persecution. Because of Dinly's embrace of "peculiar religious notions," as historian Bernhard Weinberger called them, he was disfranchised and denounced as a heretic.

During a violent storm in the winter of 1638, Dinly was sent for by a Roxbury man to perform a tooth-drawing. He and the maid who'd come to fetch him lost their way and both froze to death. Their bodies were found several days later. Dinly is thus the first barber-surgeon in the United States to lose his life in the line of duty. Perhaps it was on that white and stormy night that the venerable medical tradition of the house call began to wane. Shortly after his death, Dinly's wife gave birth to a son, christened Fathergone Dinly.

As Dinly and his untreated supplicant learned, the climate would prove less than hospitable for both dentists and their patients. In the words of one historian, the colonies "failed to provide a fertile ground for the medical profession." Those who did seek treatment were often the worse for it. Up to the 1700s, accounts claim three to seven barber-surgeons practiced in Massachusetts. Mercury was their treatment of choice; and as a result patients lost more teeth than necessary—sometimes all of them. One edentulous patient, a poor carpenter, offered to pay his fee for treatment in hay rakes, a deal his health-care provider accepted. The carpenter made them of green timber, and after a few days in the sun, all the teeth fell out—just as his had.

Other treatment protocols imported from England included this painful advice printed in 1672: "Picking the gums with the bill of an osprey is good for the toothache, and scarifying the gums with a thorn from the back of a dog fish will cure toothache."

Foul Teeth and a Free Press

NEWSPAPERS, WHICH PLAYED so large a role in early American history as clarions of colonial causes, were also integral to dentistry. Advertisements promoted the services of proto-practitioners, leaving a rich record of our dental roots. What is remarkable is the degree to which American history and American dentistry would be inextricably linked.

One influential paper was the *New York Weekly Journal*, Gotham's first, published by pioneer New World newsman John Peter Zenger (1697–1746). Trained as a printer, Zenger delighted in his role as editor and self-appointed rabble-rouser after acquiring the publication in 1733. He brought, rather than any literary sensibility, a dogged antiroyalism to its pages, using it as a platform for attacking the policies and person of New York's greedy, grubby Governor William Cosby. It was in this regard that foul teeth came to play a pivotal role in defining freedom of the press in the colonies.

Zenger's numerous critical items about Cosby included an attack on his oral hygiene. He claimed the governor had an unclean mouth and loathsome false teeth. Furious, Cosby had Zenger jailed for seditious libel. Eminent attorney Alexander Hamilton came from Philadelphia to defend Zenger, successfully arguing the article was not libelous unless the Crown could prove it false. Apparently the Crown failed to achieve the burden of proof, for Zenger was acquitted, providing the first victory for freedom of the press in the colonies and establishing an important precedent against judicial tyranny.

Wigged-Out Dentistry

THE FIRST TOOTH-DRAWER in the colonies known by name was James Reading. Like Dinly, his demise paved the way for history's recognition. We know of his practice only from a posthumous notice in the *Weekly Journal*, in 1735:

> Teeth drawn, and old broken Stumps taken out very safely and with much ease by James Mills, who was instructed in the Art by the late James Reading, deceased, so fam'd for drawing of Teeth, he is to be spoke with at his Shop in the House of the deceased, near the old Slip Market.

Mills was Reading's brother-in-law; his sister was the Prime Remover's widow. But it was not in-lawship alone that enabled Mills to take over the deceased's practice. Mills was a wig-maker, and dentistry was a common sideline for many in this field. As dental historian Max Geshwind noted, "the history of the colonial peruke-maker is also the history of the tooth-drawer of the time."

Colonial wig- or peruke-makers evolved from barbers, who were obviously familiar with hair. When wigs took the colonial fashion world by storm, barbers were well positioned to take advantage of the demand. Thus, providers of perukes also bled clients and drew teeth.

The wig, though worn from Egyptian times, came back into vogue when Louis XIII took to wearing them in 1624. The Sun King, Louis XIV, did not take up the fashion until his own hair began to fall out, but once he did, the wigged-out look became all the rage at Versailles, and soon spread to other royal courts. The fashion was quick to reach the upper classes of Restoration England, and then the colonies.

Puritans opposed the use of wigs, though they did little to stop their spread, and by the beginning of the 1700s, men and women sported them without fear of prosecution. The wig-maker's art flourished. Bleeding and tooth-drawing paid far less. Invoices from the era indicate bleeding cost about two shillings and six pence, and tooth-drawing might fetch only half that. Wig-work, however, usually started at ten shillings, and a new wig could cost several pounds.

In Williamsburg, the restored colonial village in Virginia, the tools of the trade can be seen at the Kings Arms Barber Shop, which displays artifacts of the town's wig-makers' dental practice.

Wig-workers were not the only tradesmen who practiced dentistry on the side, or "assumed the role" of dentist, as the arrival of a thespian dentist from London attests in this ad from Boston's *Independent Chronicle and Universal Advertiser* of 1799:

> C. E. Whitlock, Dentist, Respectfully acquaints the Public that his engagements at the Theatre having expired, he is now at liberty to offer his services in the above profession, to which he has been regularly bred.

Whitlock, who achieved considerable repute onstage, had been practicing dentistry in conjunction with his performing career in the United States as early as 1793, one of a circle of actor-dentists. Their ranks included famed French actor Jean Baptiste, whose repute eclipsed that of his father, Pierre Fauchard, sire of dentistry. The noted French drama star J. Talma was another.

The French Correction

COLONISTS WERE AS impressed by operators of French extraction as the British. The first such practitioner known to visit America was

French-trained dentist Sieur Roquet. He arrived in Boston in 1749 late of Paris, advertising and enumerating his services in the *Independent Advertiser* on July 3 of that year:

> ... He also cures effectually the most stinking Breaths by drawing out, and eradicating all decayed Teeth and Stumps, and burning the Gums to the Jaw Bone, without the least Pain or Confinement; and putting in their stead, an entire Set of right African Ivory Teeth, set in a Rose-colour'd Enamel, so nicely fitted to the Jaws, that People of the first Fashion may eat, drink, swear, talk, Scandal, quarrel, and shew their Teeth, without the least Indecency, Inconvenience, or Hesitation whatever. He deals only for ready Money with the Quality and Members of Parliament, but will give reasonable Credit to Citizens, Tradesmen, and Gentlemen of the Inns of Court."

Michael Poree, Operator for the Teeth, arrived from Paris in 1768, taking up residence in New York, and authoring the first lay article on dentistry written by a dentist in the Americas. It appeared in the *New York Gazette* and the *Weekly Mercury* in 1769, and included his attack on a prevalent variety of native practitioners:

> There are many erroneous operators for the teeth, who believe, and frankly confess the operation to be dangerous, yet dare to undertake it, particularly to fasten the teeth that are loose, to fill up the decay'd ones, and prevent them from aching any more, and to polish the same, and make them equal to the sound ones in strength and service and sight. But the Daily, and just exclamations of these ladies and gentlemen who have had the misfortune to suffer the most excruciating pain under such operators, and the exorbitant prices thereof, will sufficiently evince to the public, that all such operators are, in a word, worse than pick-pockets or thieves; For a person had much better lose a little money, or an handkerchief, than their teeth at any time because the former will not do, and supply the many unspeakable uses and services of the latter; for many of these operators have, by their operations, spoiled the whole set of teeth.

In recalling "the many honourable mouths I have had the honour to put in order," Poree elaborated on his belief that the teeth were of vital importance in regulating digestion, owing to their ability to control oral air flow. Thus, dental problems could hamper the mouth's ability "to receive and remit at sundry times the air which is the pendulum of life, by which we move; which must work regularly, otherwise we are disordered, and sickness ensues, which is often the case when there is a gap in the teeth, because the air goes in and out too fast, which disorders the stomach."

Another Frenchman, Dr. Dubuke, a "London occulist and Dentist" who expressed himself "glad to undertake the cure of many diseases, among them cancer," achieved such notoriety that he didn't even have to place advertisements to receive notice in the news. His movements were reported by *New York's Constitutional Gazette* in 1776:

The famous Dr. Dubuke, a Frenchman, who was branded here last January term, for stealing indigo, etc., departed last Thursday from this city in the Amboy state boat, to visit Philadelphia and the Southern Colonies. He professes himself a dentist, and has travelled through the Eastern Colonies under various names.

The British Are Coming

ANOTHER OLD WORLD practitioner, Robert Wooffendale (also spelled *Woofendale*), arrived from England in 1766. His credentials, as touted in an ad in the *New York Mercury*, were impeccable:

Robert Wooffendale
Surgeon Dentist, lately arrived from London, (who was instructed by Thomas Berdmore, Esq; Operator for the Teeth to his present Britanick Majesty) begs leave to inform the Public, that he performs all Operations upon the Teeth, Gums, Sockets, and palate: Likewise fixes artificial Teeth so as to escape Discernment, and without Pain, or the least inconvenience.
                                                —Nov. 13, 1766

Despite his pedigree, Wooffendale's practice failed to thrive in the colonies, and he returned to England in 1768, setting up an apothecary shop in Sheffield. As for his instruction from Berdmore, the esteemed dentist himself answered those claims in an ad in England's *York Courant* in 1773:

MR. BERDMORE is very sorry the imprudence of Mr. Wooffendale obliges him, in his own Vindication, to take the least notice of him in a News Paper. Mr. Berdmore wishes not to prejudice the young Man in the Opinion of such as may be inclined to employ him, but he cannot suffer the Sanction of his Name to be disingenuously imposed upon them. Mr. Wooffendale some Years ago was taken from a Druggist's Shop (to which Business he was brought up) by Mr. Berdmore, at a Salary of 25 1. per Ann. and at the Expiration of seven Years was to have been admitted to a small share of his Business; and in order to secure his Services, as it was supposed he might then be competently qualified in the Profession, he was bound in a Bond of £1000. not to practice in London; but either not liking the Confinement, or proposing some greater Advantage, he thought it fit to remove himself to America in less than six Months, during which Time he was employed in cutting Bone (ivory), and other trifling Offices. This is the plain State of the Matter. And now whether Mr. Wooffendale be, as he professes, amply qualified as a Dentist or not, Mr. Berdmore only desires it may be understood that he cannot be so from any Instructions received under him.

Rather than admit his own misrepresentations, Wooffendale, who returned to America in 1793, apparently preferred casting aspersions on others. A booklet he wrote, "Practical Observations on the Human Teeth," draped this effort in the cloak of selfless service to the unenlightened:

I am aware that, by making public the various circumstances relating to the teeth, and the operations to be performed on them, and of exposing some of the impositions and deceptions too often used, I shall draw upon myself the malevolence of

ignorant pretenders to the dentist's art. To these I have nothing
to say. Men of that profession, of liberal minds, will not want
an apology: as exposing the various mean use for imposture in
the profession, appears the most likely method of fixing it on a
more solid and liberal foundation, than has yet been done.

The exposé-cum-instructional manual would become a staple of
the communiqués by which dentists promoted their services and den-
igrated their competitors. A century later, in 1877, early dental historian Alfred Hill summed up the character of such authors and their
pronouncements:

They draw over their own ink-stained fingers the whitest of kid-
gloves, and with lifted shoulders and outstretched arms implore
the deluded, but patiently enduring, outside world to remember
that they are the only individuals capable of taking care of its
interests, so far as the teeth are concerned, at the least, and
how delighted they will be to become the fortunate deliverers
of the prey from the spoiler.

Yet even as some practitioners proclaimed their Old World training, a declaration of independence from the European tradition can be
read between the lines of an ad in the *New York Mercury* placed by
James Daniel in 1766. The ad describes Daniel as a "Wig-maker and
Hairdresser and also an operator for the teeth." From a historical perspective, his eschewment of the more popular French derivative terms
"peruke-maker and dentist," as well as the more archaic barber and
tooth-drawer, is revealing. Clearly dental professionals, as well as the
colonies, were struggling to find an identity of their own. Both would
have to endure bloodshed to claim it.

Quacks of the sort who infested London at the time also plied their
trade in the colonies. The following ad, placed in the *Virginia Gazette*
in 1768 by one "Philodontalkikos," offers a taste of their imprecations:

The subscriber, late from Constantinople, begs leave to inform
the public, that for the sole benefit of his countrymen he has
made himself acquainted with the celebrated method of ex-

tracting sound teeth, as practiced with universal success, by Mustapah Ben Achmet, great dentist to the Grand Signior, on whose certificate the subscriber offers his service.

That every man has the seeds of the tooth ach in his composition, which tho' latent for a while, will in the end, certainly discover themselves, and increase to their appointed maturity, is a position no one can question. That the teeth are the nidus of these seeds, is also unquestionable. It follows from hence, that extracting the sound teeth is laying the hand to the root of this disorder. . . . How dreadful a disorder the tooth ach is, how uncertain in its attacks and excruciating in its effects, can be unknown to few; which makes him expect that this method of removing the danger by precaution, will be universally embraced. Should this relentless malady invade an epicure in times of feasting, fine Lady dressed for a birth night, should its sudden attack pillage the beauty of a triumphant fair at a ball; or should it seize upon a bridegroom on his nuptial night, how terrible were the consequences! Think of this, O ye people, and have your teeth forthwith extracted! . . .

A Baker Treats Teeth

AS THE 1700s progressed, increasing numbers of professionally trained dentists were relocating to the colonies. Yet the first true English-trained dentist in the New World was practicing in Boston even before Robert Wooffendale's first trip to the colonies. He was John Baker, MD, and would become among the most esteemed of these transplants.

Baker arrived in the latter 1760s from County Cork, Ireland. The first evidence we have of his presence on American shores comes in the form of a farewell, printed in the *Boston Evening Post* in 1767:

John Baker
Surgeon, Dentist
  Begs leave to take this method of informing the Public, That he shall leave this Place in Twenty Days at farthest—That those who are disposed to apply to him may not be disappointed.

He also begs leave to express his Gratitude for the Favours he has received while is Boston; and hopes that those who doubted of the Safety of his Art, from its Novelty in this Country, are now convinced of its Utility and Usefulness.

Until he leaves this town he continues at Mr. Joshua Brackett's in School Street; where he will be ready to contribute to the utmost of his Power to serve the Publick In his Profession.

His Dentifrice, with proper directions for preserving the Teeth & Gums, will be to be had at Mrs. Eustis's, near the Town House, after he has left the Town. N.B. Each Pot is sealed with his Coat of Arms, as in the Margin of the Directions, to prevent Fraud.

The dentifrice he referred to was Baker's Antiscorbutic Dentifrice, "a certain Cure for all Disorders of the Teeth, Gums, and foul Breath." Americans could also choose from similar products, such as Perkins' Specific Dentifrice, Greenough's Tincture for the Gums and Toothache, and Pearl Dentifrice.

Baker's subsequent peregrinations from Boston, to New York, to Williamsburg and on to Annapolis can be traced in advertisements covering two decades, until the type ran cold in 1786. He would become successful, affluent, a prominent horseman. Yet surely when he penned the advertisement he was aware of the growing depth of anti-British sentiment swirling about America. Whereas Berdmore, in his published notices a year before, had invoked both England and the Crown (and his business had subsequently failed), Baker was apt to remain silent on his eminently respectable resumé. Even the vague reference to his nonnative background in the preceding ad disappeared when he placed the following notice in the *Virginia Gazette* in 1771 and 1772:

He cures the SCURVY in the GUMS, be it ever so bad; first cleans and scales the Teeth from the corrosive, tartarous, gritty Substance which hinders the Gums from growing, infects the Breath, and is one of the principal Causes of the Scurvy, which, if not timely prevented, eats away the Gums, so that many Peoples Teeth fall out fresh. He prevents Teeth from growing rotten, keeps such as are decayed from becoming worse, even to old Age, makes the Gums grow up from the Teeth, and renders them white and beautiful. He fills up, with Lead or Gold, those that are hollow, so as to render them useful; it prevents the Air from getting into them, which aggravates the Pain. He transplants natural Teeth from one Person to another, which will be as firm in the jaw as . . . [those which] originally grew there. . . . He makes and fixes artificial Teeth with the greatest Exactness and Nicety, without Pain or the least Inconvenience, so that they may eat, drink, or sleep, with them in the Mouth as natural Ones, from which they cannot be discovered by the sharpest Eye. He displaces Teeth and Stumps, after the best and easiest Methods, be they ever so deep sunk into the Socket of the Gums.

Baker's home in Williamsburg, now restored, contains a ledger documenting the financial aspects of his practice with records of payments and services rendered. Although we cannot say definitively George Washington slept here, we can say the future Father of his country had dental work done on the premises, submitting to treatment in 1772, 1773, and 1774. (A William Baker also attended to Washington's teeth occasionally, though John's services were evidently preferred.) Baker's influence on American history can be argued to go beyond dentistry, even beyond Washington's mouth, owing to his influence on another colonial hero whom he mentored in Boston, the heart of America's cradle of sedition.

A Revered Dentist

ALTHOUGH THERE IS no record of Baker's arrival in Beantown, by his own estimate he had treated "upward of 2,000 persons in the town of Boston" by the time he decamped for New York. He had also endeavored to train a local craftsman as his replacement. It was a mantle the trainee felt sufficiently comfortable wearing to place his own ad in both the *Boston News Letter* and the *Boston Gazette* and *Country Journal* in August of the following year, 1768:

Whereas many persons are so unfortunate as to lose their Fore-Teeth by Accident, and otherways, to their great Detriment, not only in Looks, but speaking both in Public and Private:—This is to inform all such, that they may have them re-placed with artificial Ones, that looks as well as the Natural, & answers the End of Speaking to all Intents, by PAUL REVERE, Goldsmith, near the Head of Dr. Clarke's Wharf, Boston.

All Persons who have had false Teeth fixt by Mr. John Baker, Surgeon-Dentist, and they have got loose (as they will in Time) may have them fastened by the above, who learnt the Method of fixing them from Mr. Baker.

It is for his exploits as a silversmith, engraver, and patriot that Revere is best remembered today. But one can infer from the following ad, which first appeared in the *Boston Gazette* of June 30, 1770, that he was known to most of his contemporaries as a dentist:

Artificial-Teeth
   Paul Revere,
   Takes this method of turning his most sincere Thanks to the Gentlemen and Ladies who have employed him in the care of their Teeth, he would now inform them and all others, who are so unfortunate as to lose their Teeth by accident or otherwise, that he still continues the Business of a Dentist, and flatter himself that from the Experience he has had these Two Years (in which time he has fixt some Hundreds of Teeth) that he can fix them as well as any Surgeon, Dentist who ever came from London, he fixes them in such a Manner that they are not only an Ornament but of real use in Speaking and Eating: He cleans the Teeth and will wait on any Gentleman or Lady at the Lodgings, he may be spoke with at his Shop opposite Dr. Clark's at the North-End, where the Gold and Silversmith's Business is carried on in all its Branches.

Given the rectitude of our founding fathers we can regard the copy points in this ad as factual, and certainly the claim of having fixed hundreds of teeth isn't hard to accept, considering one complete set consists of over a score and a half. What intrigues is the ad's subtext of rising tension that would result in armed insurrection just six years later. Revere's claim to have acquired, in two years, experience which enabled him to fix teeth "as well as any Surgeon, Dentist who ever came from London" demonstrates the brazenness, native confidence, cockiness, and animosity that would play itself out in the American Revolution.

At the very least, this ad can be read as a slap in the face of his mentor. Surely this latent hostility was not at variance with public sentiment of the time, and no doubt struck a responsive chord with many potential customers. Some could argue the royalist-baiting subtext was no more than a clever advertising ploy. Whatever the impetus for the brash tone, this appears to be the last ad Revere placed for his dental practice, though the same ad appeared in July and August of 1770.

Entries in Revere's diary indicate he continued practicing dentistry until 1774. It can hardly go unremarked that this is the year prior to his famed midnight ride. One must wonder to what degree the practice of dentistry allowed Revere to sublimate his animus toward England. To what extent did it provide a feeling of empowerment, a tangible way to demonstrate his (and by extension his countrymen's) equality with the English? In what way did the abandonment of this practice contribute to his involvement in revolutionary activities?

A Revolution in Forensics

THOUGH HE ABANDONED dentistry, Revere continued making bridges and dentures. In 1775 he constructed a bridge of hippopotamus ivory to replace missing teeth for his friend Dr. Joseph Warren, a noted physician and leader of colonial rebels, affixing them in place with silver wire. When hostilities commenced, Warren was commissioned as a general in the Massachusetts Militia. The enjoyment of his rank and new dental bridge would be short-lived. Among the first to give his life in the Revolution, General Warren was killed at the Battle of Bunker Hill. The dead received a hasty burial necessitated by the British advance. The common grave was left unmarked, perhaps to protect the deceased from both the British and the "ghoulish vandals," as one historian called them, referring to the scavengers who extracted teeth on battlefields for sale to dentists for dentures.

Their resting place was apparently not sufficiently camouflaged. Captain Laurie of the British forces reported he found Warren's body and "stuffed the scoundrel with another Rebel into one hole and there he and his seditious principles may remain."

A year later, with the battlefield again under colonial control, the citizens of Massachusetts sought to rebury the general with the honor he deserved. The grave site was located, the bodies exhumed, but decomposition made positive identification impossible. Several of the unearthed remains fit Warren's description. While officials tried to determine which were the war hero's, the public grew restive, criticizing the year-long delay to retrieve the "distinguished patriot" and their inability to identify his body.

Finally, Revere offered to attempt to identify the general from his bridgework. He accompanied a committee to Bunker Hill, viewed the gathered remains, found his handiwork, and made a positive ID on General Warren's body. The event was noted by the *New England Chronicle* of April 25, 1776:

> Though the body which our savage enemies scarce privileged with earth enough to hide it from the birds of prey, was disfigured, when taken up, yet it was sufficiently known by two artificial teeth, which were set for him a short time before his glorious exit."

Metaphorically, it could be said the device was a rude bridge that arched a flood. The general received his hero's burial and Revere received credit as a pioneer forensic odontologist, having made what is believed to be the first identification of human remains by teeth in the Americas.

Revere's mentor, Dr. Baker, continued to enjoy success in America, both during and after the Revolution. We can infer this not only from his own advertising, but from notices such as the following, placed by a patient of Philip Clumberg, a Philadelphia barber and toothdrawer, in the *Freeman's Journal* in 1784:

> Let me seriously advise you to lay aside the performance (if you so call it) Of tooth drawing, as you have this day done me great injury in your attempt, or I would say barbarous and violent exertion. Indeed the consequences of the fracture you have produced in my jaw and the quantity of Gums and flesh

torn away by your instrument and fingers is not and will not be known for some days. Dr. Baker has just left me, after extracting the splinters of bone you occasioned. I expect every moment to spit out the two sound teeth you have displayed.

Yours, etc.,

John Felsted, The corner of Third and Vine streets.

Native Species

A NATIVE SPECIES of dentists evolved as the young nation did. Dr. Benjamin Fendall, among the first of note, was active from the 1770s to early in the 1800s. Barely a month after the signing of the Declaration of Independence, he made a stirring declaration of his own in the *Maryland Gazette* of August 15, 1776:

The oratory of the pulpit and bar, and above all the art of pleasing in conversation and social life, are matters of the highest concern to individuals. But in these no one can excel whose loss of teeth, or rotten livid stumps, and fallen lips and hollow cheeks, destroy articulation, and the happy expression of countenance; whose voice has lost its native tone, and whose laugh, instead of painting joy and merriment, expresses only defect and disease.

The foulness of the teeth by some people is little regarded; but with the fair sex, with the polite and elegant part of the world, it is looked on as a certain mark of filthiness and sloth; not only because it disfigures one of the greatest ornaments of the countenance, but also because the smell imparted to the breath by dirty rotten teeth, is generally disagreeable to the patients themselves, and sometimes extremely offensive to the olfactory nerves in close conversation.

The extent of Fendall's professional activities are difficult to ascertain, even his first name hard to verify. He is, however, the same B. Fendall who we will later see provided such poor prosthetic service to Mrs. George Washington in the last years of the century. A prolific advertiser, Fendall's copy-intensive entreaties often reached a foot in length, packed with dense type. The text revealed a sophisticated understanding of the nature of teeth and their disorders. Given Fendall's lack of professional training, any surprise this provokes must be tempered with the realization the ads are copied almost-verbatim from Thomas Berdmore's dental opus.

Yanking Ingenuity

YANKEE INGENUITY was now making itself felt in American dentistry. James Gardette (1756–1831) of Philadelphia, often called the first medically trained dentist to practice in America, substituted elastic flat gold bands, or braces, in place of traditional ligatures of silk or fine gold wire used to secure artificial teeth. As we will see, he also would be responsible for major advances in prosthetic devices, and provided dental services to George Washington (as did most leading dentists of the day).

In 1797, the first United States patent for a dental device was granted to Thomas Bruff for a "perpendicular extractor." Whether this represented an actual advance is questionable. He advised potential patients "that the pain of this mode of extracting . . . is not to be regarded by the most delicate persons." He quickly sold off the rights to its use in Baltimore, where he practiced, and in a subsequent ad in the *Maryland Journal,* informed anyone needing an extraction he was "fully prepared to perform the operation with the greatest care"—except cases requiring the use of his patented Perpendicular Extractor.

Traveling, or itinerant dentists, were a staple of early American oral care. Roaming throughout their territory, they would announce their impending arrival in a town in newspapers, posters, and handbills like the following: "Tooth extracted absolutely without pain by the use of Odonto, the only local anesthetic known which makes the extraction of all teeth, sore or otherwise, absolutely painless, and leaves no after effect in any case," claimed a poster for "Painless Dentistry" practiced by H. H. Barnard. "Persons suffering with heart or lung disease can have teeth extracted by its use with perfect safety. There's no more danger in having 32 teeth extracted than one or two in one sitting."

As a caveat, it added: "Caution, be aware of all persons claiming to use this preparation as it is manufactured and used only by H. H. Barnard of Millford, New York. Odonto."

Upon arrival, the itinerant dentist would set up shop in a hotel room or outdoors in the town square. He traveled light. A portable headrest was clamped to the back of a chair, the small leather bag of tools was opened, and the itinerant was ready to go to work. As long as people showed up, the dentist remained rooted. When volume thinned, they moved on. Even the most successful dentists periodically decamped to ply their trade in other cities. This was not an exclusively male fraternity, either. Mrs. Dodge of New York, the first female itinerant dentist, is known to have hit the road in 1797, demonstrating her "art dental" to the ladies of Boston and vicinity.

For training, American dentists by and large shunned book-learning. There were no reference manuals or tomes they ever "depended on for substance and inspiration," in the words of one historian, save Hunter's *Natural History of the Human Teeth*. By the time its supplement, *A Practical Treatise on the Diseases of the Teeth*, appeared in 1778, the former colonies and England were no longer on speaking terms. But the skirmish of flesh and din of muskets failed to blunt the ongoing battle for this book, and the two volumes ultimately had a profound influence on the practice of dentistry in the United States.

But much of the population had no access to professional dentists—qualified or otherwise. When a dental emergency arose, they had to make do with the tools and tradesmen at hand. The historical novel *One Red Rose Forever*, set among the Pennsylvania Dutch settlers of Lancaster County, Pennsylvania, in 1769, offers a rather graphic account of one such tooth extraction, performed by a country barber using a hammer and nail.

Whether because of such care or lack of it, colonists exhibited poor oral health. One traveler disdainfully reported, "Men and women . . . lose their teeth: the woman are pitifully Tooth-shaken; whether through the coldness of the climate or the sweetmeats . . . I'm not able to affirm. . . ."

Oral neglect and its consequences were obvious even in civilized areas. In private correspondence between a pair of sisters from Long Island in 1781, the writer describes a young, carious acquaintance as a symbol of her generation: "Her teeth are beginning to decay, which is the case with most New York girls, after eighteen."

War of Words

THE END OF the American Revolution did not signal the cessation of hostilities for all dentist-combatants. One brutal campaign embroiled dentist Josiah Flagg (1763–1816), and put Thomas Paine on the firing line.

Born in Boston in 1764, Flagg was the son of a lieutenant colonel in the in Continental Army, and was said to have risen to the rank of major during the war. Where he received his dental training is unclear. His father and Paul Revere were friends, having copublished songs as early as 1765, and perhaps Flagg could have acquired some instruction from Revere. Reference is made to training received from a French officer during the Revolution, but whether Flagg actually served in the war is also unclear.

He began practicing dentistry around 1783. Something of a showboater, historians allege he may have frequently exaggerated his claims, standard operating procedure in those times. In 1795, for example, he announced the availability of his patent "artificial teeth of China enamel." An examination of patent office records finds no such patent on file, though one for "Lamps, reflectors, Elastic," was granted to Flagg and his son fifteen years later.

One of the first colonial oral surgeons, among the repairs his ads listed him capable were "sews up hare-lips and fixes gold roofs and palates, greatly assisting the pronunciation and the swallow."

His inflated claims and arrogant advertising (one began "DR. FLAGG, continues his Practice, as SURGEON DENTIST the most successful of the profession, in all its branches . . .") led to a bitter rivalry with William Pitt Greenwood (1766–1851), a renowned dentist who performed a great variety of operations. Greenwood lost no opportunity to impugn Flagg's credentials, attacks which possibly drove Flagg out of practice in 1792.

In 1795 Flagg placed an advertisement in the *Federal Orrery* of Boston, announcing his "return to practice as a surgeon dentist." Three days later, the paper's editor, Thomas Paine planted the following item in the paper:

A correspondent is happy to find DR. FLAGG has returned to Boston. He hopes that his old enemies will now be ashamed of

their groundless malice, and that the Dr. will resume his practice, with his former emolument and reputation.

Paine's support for Flagg arose perhaps out of regard for his father's
wartime service, or perhaps because he was an advertiser. Any conflict
of interest, any breach between the paper's advertising and editorial
departments went unremarked. But Flagg's return didn't. In an ad the
following year Flagg proclaimed:

> He is sorry thus publicly to observe, that some illiberal and
> unjust insinuations have been propagated, to bias the minds of
> individuals, and give a false colouring to his professional rep-
> utation. Those good-natured people have even ventured so far
> to say, that undue advantage has been taken on those who have
> appealed for his assistance, by extorting from them, a sum be-
> yond the bounds of their expectation.
>   To confute any of the like slander in future, he declares that
> his fees may be always known previous to his operating, and
> the person at free liberty to employ him or seek assistance
> elsewhere.

During the War of 1812, Flagg enlisted in the navy but was soon
captured and remanded to London, where he practiced dentistry for
the duration. Returning to America following the war, he was ship-
wrecked in New York harbor. In poor health from his exposure, the
decision was made to repair to the warmer clime of Charleston, South
Carolina. However, a few days after his arrival, he contracted yellow
fever and died. His sons would carry on the name in dentistry, and the
family played an important role in its progress for over a century.

Flagg's nemesis, William Pitt Greenwood, was himself a member
of one of early America's most acclaimed dental dynasties, founded by
Isaac Greenwood Sr. (1730–1803). Isaac senior entered the business
as a sideline to his primary occupation as an umbrella maker and ivory
turner, or carver. Four of his sons—Isaac Jr., John, Clark, and William
Pitt—became well-known dentists. Adding confusing to the array of
Greenwoods were the third-generation dentists, including John's two
sons, Isaac John and Clark.

Isaac senior's son John may have been the first dentist to use a foot
drill. According to an account provided by his son Isaac John, years

later, "he made it himself from an old spinning wheel of my grand-mother's; and, since his death I myself used it, the same one, altogether in my practice for twenty years, and have it yet. I never had seen one before, and I know the hand bow-drill was always used before."

When Isaac junior began practicing, he was anxious to burnish his father's reputation and perhaps advance the family's dynastic ambitions. In an ad in New York's *Weekly Museum* in 1792, he stated his father, from whom he'd acquired his skills, "is well known to be eminent in the line of that profession now and for thirty years past."

Most people reading the ad probably didn't check the facts, but historians have. Greenwood senior's primary business before 1780, is clear: "Umbrilloes made and Sold by Isaac Greenwood, Turner at his Shop in Forest Street. . . ." began one in the *Boston Gazette and Country Journal* in 1769. No mention of dental services is made.

Greenwood senior turned his attention to drawing teeth and making dentures in about 1778. Though he apparently never expanded his abilities beyond dentures and extractions, he achieved great success. Yet all his ads reference his occupation as ivory turner and umbrella maker.

He is credited as being the first to mount a public-education advertising campaign and, more important, the first practitioner to adopt a dental slogan. In promoting a health-care ménage à trois of sorts, an open relationship involving a dentist, a patient, and a physician, he coined the tag line, "Advise with your physician."

5

A New Era in Teethpulling

Anesthetics Usher in Painless Dentistry

PAIN AND DENTISTRY LONG ENDURED A CRUEL SYMBIOSIS, A throbbing bond formed at the exposed ends of man's most sensitive nerves. Today we are fortunate to live in the golden era of "painless" dentistry, a sensorially attenuated epoch mankind has struggled for millennia to reach.

A Natural High

THE ANCIENTS GATHERED anesthetics from nature. They discovered plants whose extracts could dull or alter the senses, and concocted potions from their roots and leaves. Pyrethrum and mandrake root (a member of the nightshade family) were popular around the Mediterranean region. Wine mixed with mandragora (a mandrake concoction) was another common anesthetic. Hyoscyamine, or henbane, and ivy and hemlock were also used. In the Middle East and the Orient, opium was the painkiller of choice. Hashish was also used in the Middle East while early Chinese physicians sometimes prescribed marijuana and employed acupuncture to dull pain during operations. Pien Chico, a Chinese practitioner who lived about 300 B.C., wrote of an Eastern anesthetic that seems remarkably advanced even by today's standards:

> Two men by the name of Lu and Chao visited me. I gave them
> a subtle drink which reduced them to unconsciousness for three
> whole days. Then I operated on them and explored the regions
> of the stomach and the heart. I then cut out both heart and
> stomach and exchanged them in these two persons. Such was

the wonderful drug that they uttered no sound and in a few days I suffered them to return home fully recovered.

The Story of O

As PIEN CHICO suggests, the development of surgery provided an impetus for finding an effective painkiller. The first record of a surgical operation uncovered thus far is on an Egyptian bas-relief dating from about 4000 B.C. It depicts the circumcision of a boy at puberty. A woman restrains the young man's hands while before him kneels the priest, ready to begin trimming the foreskin. From the terror etched in the youngster's face, we can infer no anesthetic has been applied.

Egyptians would later blunt their pain with opium. Opium poppies are discussed among the 700 remedies listed in the Papyrus Ebers. Hailed as a gift of the gods, its discovery was described in Egyptian mythology:

> The great Sun-God Ra called on the Goddess Tefnut to cure the terrible pains he endured. Beautiful Tefnut was not skilled in the art of medicine and the concoction she gave her master produced a terrible headache. But pitying Isis brought juice from the 'berry-of-the-poppy plant' and Ra was instantly cured.

Opium may have been known to the Greeks as well. In the *Odyssey*, Homer refers to a mind-numbing drug called nepenthe dispensed by Helen: "Presently she cast a drug in to the wine whereof they drank, a drug to lull all pain and anger and bring forgetfulness of every sorrow."

The active ingredient remained unidentified, though some have speculated if such a narcotic existed, it may have been a form of purified opium.

Pain was a major medical concern of the Greeks. When the shrines of Aesculapius at Kos and Epidaurus were uncovered, a bizarre collection of stone and iron replicas of faces contorted in pain, along with innumerable prayers describing the miseries that prompted these expressions (and the relief Aesculapius subsequently granted them) were found.

Hippocrates was greatly interested in alleviating pain, and used ice and snow to numb limbs for operations. Witnessing the death of Socrates provoked a sophisticated analysis of the subject:

> The hemlock which Socrates took that sent him on his journey to God, that hemlock holds the secret to our search. . . . It induces sleep, and a paralysis of the nether limbs. I remember that when this poison had nearly completed its work, Socrates, in order to test how far death stood from him, put his hand to his mouth and bit it. I watched his face closely and could recognize no pain. Now, you may think it wrong that I should notice such details on the death-bed of the great, but Socrates, who loved his fellow men, would have wished it so. If we could so distill hemlock that we could rid it of its death-giving propensities, we may find the answer to the riddle we seek.

Becoming Unnerved

ROMANS EXPERIMENTED WITH pain eradication as well, sometimes with lethal results. One recommended method called for bringing pressure to the great carotid arteries in the neck, thereby diminishing the blood flow and inducing unconsciousness. In some unfortunate cases, the brain ceased functioning altogether.

Galen killed pain during extractions by applying pickled root of pyrethrum, or chrysanthemum, to the teeth and gum. The corrosive concoction, in addition to deadening pain, probably partially destroyed and loosened the periodontal membrane and attachment fibers holding the tooth in place. Such was its power that neighboring teeth were shielded by a coating of wax to prevent unnecessary tooth loss. Galen reported he could perform extractions using his bare fingers following the application.

Mandrake was one of the empire's primary painkillers, and was the main ingredient of a nerve-deadening soporific similar to Galen's, popular during the reign of Nero. Pliny, archivist of misinformation, wrote that mandrake grew in both male and female varieties, erroneous assertions carried forward after the fall of Rome. Thus, medieval mandrake hunters were warned against the terrible scream the plants would make when picked. It was advised that to capture the mandrake, hunters should "Stuff the ears with good bees' wax. Sift the earth around the mandrake and then attach a long piece of string to a dog's tail. See that this dog is either ailing or at the most very small and worthless. Then tie the other end of the string to the mandrake, give sharp kick in the wretched cur' loins. As the creature jumps forward, the root will give its dreadful cry and the dog instead of a man will go mad or drop dead."

Pliny also wrote of a mystic *Lapis memphitis,* or stone of Memphis. It supposedly worked as a local anesthetic when rubbed on the surface of the skin in conjunction with sour wine.

Pain hardly subsided with the fall of Rome, but advances in anesthetics did. Other than the inclusion of worthless additives, state-of-the-art anesthetics at the end of the first millennium were no better than the Romans'. A commonly prescribed anodyne—a pain-relieving potion or talisman—of the era combined opium, celandine (a member of the poppy family), and saffron with oil of lizards, bone marrow, and the fat of man.

As Europe awoke from its medieval torpor, new methods of sensory deprivation were developed. In 1220 Hugo de Lucca introduced *spongia somnifera,* or sleep sponges. They were prepared by soaking sponges in a concentrated solution of opium, hemlock, henbane, mandragora, lettuce seeds, and other powerful additives, then drying them in the sun. When it came time to induce anesthesia, the sponges were soaked in hot water and applied to the nostrils. When it was time to resuscitate the patient, a sponge or cotton lint soaked in vinegar was substituted. These sponges were used by Guy de Chauliac and other surgeons of the era.

During the same age, anesthetics progressed from natural substances to man-made chemicals with the discovery of ether. Among those credited with first identifying ether are the twelfth-century Arabian chemist Yeber and the monk and alchemist Raymond Lullus (1235–1315), both of whom presumably stumbled upon it while trying to turn base metal into gold. Lullus recognized its anesthetic properties, calling it "sweet vitriol." The rest of the world remained ignorant of its potential in pain management, consequently suffering centuries of needless suffering, though hardly in silence.

Paracelsus, whom we met presiding over the book-burning in Basel, discovered the properties of ether independently in the early 1500s. Reportedly he'd mixed sulfuric acid with alcohol and was heating the mixture when a whiff of the resulting gas wafted his way, semi-sedating him into sudden realization of its potential. He later experimented on chickens and found it could induce sleep. Still the medical and dental communities ignored the promising palliative.

The medieval world had another shot at putting ether to work when it was independently discovered yet again in 1542 by Valerius Cordus, who called it *oleum vitrioli dulce*, echoing the name Lullus gave it. An English chemist dubbed it ether in 1730.

Why was ether's beneficial properties overlooked for so long? Some might suggest those inflicting rather than feeling the pain had little vested interest in its reduction. Even after ether's widespread acceptance in the late nineteenth century, some physicians opposed its use, contending the sensation of pain was a requirement for the body to survive an operation.

With no other anesthetics in the R&D pipeline, the use of cold to deaden nerves was reintroduced early in the 1600s. But for all the opium, ether, sponges, and ice, eliminating the horrific pain of an extraction remained beyond the reach of dentistry.

There was the occasional flash from the pain-fighting front, but little of substance. In 1774 Franz Anton Mesmer, an Austrian physician, introduced magnetic cures, known as Mesmerisms, into medicine. Magnets were already popular in quack remedies. Mesmer believed the true source of magnetism's therapeutic power came from within the individual. His techniques were meant to harness that inner human force. He achieved admirable success treating what we would term psychosomatic illness, but his acclaim alarmed other physicians. A committee formed by University of Vienna to investigate his methods recommended a cessation of his "fraudulent practice."

Hounded from his home country, Mesmer moved to Paris, published *Memoir on the Discovery of Animal Magnetism*, and opened a clinic in the Hotel Bullion in Rue Montmartre. The results of Mesmerism's use for pain relief during dental procedures were less than encouraging. He was ultimately discredited by a commission formed by the French government.

In 1794 a writer in Florence, Italy, reported that residents of the Tuscan countryside used certain species of beetles as a topical anesthetic for toothache, principally the ladybird, *coccionella septempunctata,* and the *curculio antiodontalgicus,* a beetle found on spiny shrubs in the area. Larvae were crushed between the fingers and the resulting pulp rubbed on the gum of the affected tooth. The insects are said to contain a substance chemically allied to cantharidin, the blistering constituent of Spanish fly, the rubefacient (an agent that causes reddening of the skin by dilating the blood vessels) made from the beetle of that name. Could this in any way hearken to Pliny's writings of a worm that lived on reeds that cured toothaches? If one considers his record for accuracy, chances are slim.

Nitrous Oxide: Ticket to Paradise

WHILE MESMERIZED DENTAL patients were using magnet and mind trying to overcome pain, the seminal discovery of the modern era of anesthesia had already been made. The man responsible was English chemist Joseph Priestly (1733–1804). Today remembered in the scientific world at large as the discoverer of what he called "dephlogisticated air"—oxygen—in dental circles he is better remembered for his 1773 discovery of "dephlogisticated nitrous air," better known as nitrous oxide or laughing gas. His surviving notebooks also recount pioneering experiments with electricity:

> I killed a pretty large kitten with the discharge of a battery of thirty-three square feet . . . I endeavoured to bring it back to life by distending the lungs, blowing with a quill into the trachea, but to no purpose.

After discovering nitrous oxide, Priestly conducted experiments with it using animals as test subjects, beginning with a pair of mice. The results of this research have been lost to history, or perhaps more accurately, to fire. Priestly, a peculiar polymath, didn't confine himself to science. A theologian and political theorist as well, he made himself remarkably unpopular in his community. One of his religious tracts was publicly burned. A political pamphlet he subsequently authored was responsible for inciting a mob to raze his house, his laboratory and books going up in flames along with the rest of it, prompting his relocation to the United States. Given the extent of his interests and his need to flee, it's not surprising he failed to continue investigating the properties of his discovery.

A young scientist, Humphrey Davy (1778–1829) assigned himself responsibility for further investigation into the properties of the vapor. He wrote of his first experiment, in which he was the research subject on January 11, 1799:

> A thrilling extending from the chest to the extremities was almost immediately produced. I felt a sense of tangible extension highly pleasurable in every limb; my visible impressions were dazzling, and apparently magnified, I heard every sound in the room, and was perfectly aware of my situation. . . . As I recovered my former state of mind I felt an inclination to communicate the discoveries I had made during the experiment. I endeavored to recall the ideas: they were feeble and indistinct.

Clearly intoxicated with the thrill of research, Davy virtually donated his body to science. Within months he had succeeded in producing pure nitrous oxide for use in his studies. The gas was pumped into silk bags, from whence it was inhaled. Davy called these silken reservoirs "Paradise bags," breathlessly writing that they "held the key to paradise." He built an elaborate breathing chamber in which to sit and inhale the vapors and documented the results in precise detail. His findings, published in 1800, created a sensation, and can be seen as a landmark work in a body of literature that would grow to include Aldous Huxley's *The Doors of Perception* and William Burroughs's *Junkie*.

Davy invited the Lake poets to participate in his experiments. Samuel Taylor Coleridge, an inveterate opium addict, took to the gas with particular passion. "I experienced the most voluptuous sensations. The outer world grew dim and I had the most entrancing visions. For three and a half minutes I lived in a world of new sensations," Coleridge rhapsodized of his Xanadu-like experience.

Another well-known contemporary drug abuser, Thomas De Quincey, blamed dental discomfort for his habit. Author of the controversial *Confessions of an English Opium Eater,* De Quincey condemned Coleridge's use of opium but forgave his own due to its genesis:

> Most truly I have told the reader, that not any search after pleasure, but mere extremity of pain from rheumatic toothache—this and nothing else it was that first drove me into the

use of opium. Coleridge's bodily affliction was simple rheumatism. Mine, which intermittently raged for ten years, was
rheumatism in the face combined with toothache.

The results of Davy's research of nitrous oxide can be summed up
succinctly: It's a gas. His self-experimentation and the imprimatur of
celebrity addicts moved the vapor out of the laboratories and into the
world of popular entertainment. Soon the effects of inhalation were
being demonstrated on stage, at public lectures, in private homes, or
anywhere proper gentlemen and ladies gathered. Audience participation was encouraged. Yet the affect for which the gas would have its
greatest application—numbing pain—remained ignored and unex-
plored, even though Davy himself had documented its efficacy in relieving toothaches:

> The power of the immediate operation of the gas in removing
> intense physical pain I had a very good opportunity of ascer-
> taining. . . . In curing one of the unlucky teeth called the *den-*
> *tes sapiente*, I experienced an extensive inflammation of the
> gum, accompanied with great pain, which equally destroyed
> the power of repose, and of consistent action. On the day
> when the inflammation was most troublesome, I breathed
> three large doses of nitrous oxide. The pain was diminished
> after the first four or five inspirations; the thrilling came on
> as usual, and uneasiness was for a few minutes swallowed up
> in pleasure.

(Sertürner, who first refined opium into morphine in 1804, used
nitrous oxide on himself for relief of a toothache.)

Davy furthered his research at a "pneumatic institute" in Clifton.
In his book *Medical Vapors* he made a startling claim for what he called
"the pleasure-producing air": "As nitrous oxide in its intensive operation appears capable of destroying physical pain, it may be used with
advantage during surgical operations in which no great effusion of
blood takes place."

But unskilled administrators helped fuel a swift and powerful backlash, and soon the use of laughing gas as an inhalant in England was
prohibited by law. Davy and the rest of society turned their backs on
the gas. Davy moved on to more conventional scientific pursuits. After

inventing a mining lamp and a new kind of gunpowder, he was knighted in 1812 and received a baronetcy in 1818.

United States Gas Attack

BY THE EARLY 1830s, audiences in the United States were being introduced to laughing gas by a contingent of itinerant lecturers, traveling showmen who toured the country delivering presentations and demonstrations created to enlighten, entertain, and acculturate the public: infotainment, in today's parlance. Whether the content of these presentations was factual or spurious was typically of no great import in this form of performance art. What mattered was providing audiences with a level of excitement and titillation similar to that provided today by tabloid newspapers.

A sense of the tenor of the times is gleaned by reading ads for these performances, such as one promoting an eighteen-year-old lad who billed himself as "Dr. S. Coult of Calcutta, London and New York," who appeared in Portland, Maine on October 13, 1832:

> *Nitrous Oxide Gas for Ladies and Gentlemen*
> Dr. S. Coult respectfully informs the Ladies and Gentlemen of Portland and vicinity, that he will administer the NITROUS OXIDE, or Exhilarating Gas, on Monday evening at the City Hall. . . . Dr. C. has exhibited the extraordinary powers of the gas in many cities of the United States, to audiences composed of Ladies and Gentlemen of the first respectability—and many ladies have inhaled the gas at select Exhibitions. Those Ladies who may be anxious of witnessing the Exhibition, in this city, may be assured, that the City Hall embraces every accommodation for their comfort, and that not a shadow of impropriety attends the Exhibition, to shock the most modest. He will attend, on reasonable terms, to any applications for private Exhibitions to select parties of Ladies and Gentlemen. . . .

With its increasing use as a recreational drug, the wonder is that its medicinal benefits, an application right under everyone's nose, remained unrecognized. Finally it fell to one Gardner Quincey Colton

(1814–1898), an itinerant lecturer working the northeast corridor, to earn posterity's honor. On the evening of December 10, 1844, Colton brought his laughing-gas exhibition to Hartford, Connecticut.

People took their nitrous straight in those days, unlike the oxygen-diluted cocktail administered by today's dentists, and its effects were much more pronounced. A few snorts, and inhalers felt no pain. From what can be inferred from Colton's account, the audience participation segment of the evening's demonstration was a smashing success. A young man by the name of Cooley became so intoxicated by the gas he began "jumping about" violently, knocking into wooden benches or settees (Colton, perhaps feeling the effects himself, was unsure which), oblivious to the injury he caused himself.

"He was astonished," Colton wrote, "to find his legs bloody, and said he did not know he had run against a bench and felt no pain after the effects of the gas had passed off."

The New Era Arrives

AMONG THE ATTENDEES who observed the incident was Horace Wells, a dentist and physician. He'd been seated next to Cooley, "noticed the circumstances" of the injury and the lack of sensation and, according to Colton, "as the audience was retiring, asked me why a man could not have a tooth extracted without pain while under the influence of the gas. I replied that I did not know, as the idea had never occurred to me. Dr. Wells then said he . . . would try it upon himself if I would bring a bag of gas to his dental office."

Wells also fired off a note to a student of his, John Riggs: "My dear John, I would appreciate it very much if you would kindly come to-morrow to my surgery and pull out one of my teeth that has been giving me a lot of trouble. I want you to come to me because I am going to experiment with a new stuff which I believe is going to numb the feeling of pain."

No crackpot, Wells had studied dentistry in Boston, though before the city's college of dentistry had been founded, and was regarded in the front ranks of local practitioners. Wells invented and made many of his own instruments.

The next morning Colton brought an inflated bladder to Wells's office and administered the gas. Riggs was given the task of the extracting the troublesome molar. The operation was quick and, most important, painless.

"A new era in teethpulling!" Wells is said to have proclaimed. "It did not hurt me more than the prick of a pin."

This was the first operation performed with modern anesthesia and the forerunner of the application of all subsequent anesthetics. Wells immediately grasped the implication and set out to bring attention to his discovery. He used nitrous oxide to perform painless dental procedures around Hartford, Connecticut. With the exception of a few near overdoses, use of the gas seemed to present no problem. Next he wrote to Dr. William Thomas Green (W. T. G.) Morton, a former student in Boston, and asked him to arrange a demonstration of the gas for the Dental Society of Boston before a class of Cambridge College Medical students at Boston General Hospital—the Big Time.

The demonstration was arranged. A young man was to be the subject for the extraction. The gas, unfortunately, was inadequately supplied. An eyewitness account provides the details of the results.

[Wells] did not reckon with the strong constitution of the student; at the same time frightened to give too much gas, because many of his patients in Hartford nearly died from inhaling more than the usual dose, Wells only gave the patient a few seconds to inhale and then applied his forceps and started pulling.

What started next was pandemonium—the patient started yelling his head off and gesticulating wildly, nearly knocking Dr. Wells on the floor. The two dentists tried vainly to restrain him, but he was too strong for them, and pushing aside the chair and instruments scattered on the floor, he went for Wells, bent on revenge for the hoax that had been played on him. And the audience followed suit. "Humbug, swindle," they shouted, "throw him out. This is a university and not a circus."

It was the beginning of a backlash that would leave nitrous oxide alternately forgotten and condemned by the American medical establishment for almost two decades. As a result of this humiliation, Wells was said to have abandoned dentistry altogether, though not his efforts to find and promote an anesthetic that would ease the suffering of the masses.

The dosage mistake was understandable. Gas was made by dentists themselves, typically filling a five-gallon rubber bag and using an ordinary hard rubber stopcock to confine the gas in the vessel. Patients inhaled from, and exhaled into the bag, eventually emptying it as they rendered themselves insensitive. There was little way to regulate the amount inspired. At one point, Thomas Crapper and Co., original manufacturers of the toilet, built a special hyperbaric chamber big enough to hold ten people for group gassing, though how the attending dentist or physician would avoid becoming intoxicated was not addressed in the design. Patient reaction to nitrous oxide was not a well-studied phenomenon, either. Dentists who experimented with it, like the itinerant lecturers, could not always be sure what behavior to expect from nitrous-giddy people. In these early days of anesthesia, dentists didn't know how to minimize the "excitement phase" of the nitrous intoxication, as dental historian Dr. Malvin Ring pointed out. Such was the perceived danger, that many dentists, even after its eventual acceptance, abandoned the use of gas due to fears of bodily harm.

The fears of possible miscues were apparently justified. In the northern peninsula of Michigan where miners, lumberers, and other brawny laborers held sway, a dentist at the dawn of the twentieth century described how he watched his mentor, whom he described as a "visionary," apply nitrous oxide. The gas was stored in an upside-down fish-tanklike contraption, over water, forced into the patients lungs via a mask.

When (the patient) was sufficiently asphyxiated, we hurriedly dropped the mask and, grabbing the forceps, got on with the job. When multiple extractions were undertaken, the patient was generally lustily kicking before the last tooth was out, so two further precautions were taken—a strong leather strap to keep the patient in the chair, and a good kicking space clear of all obstructions. Even so, the dentist often had to be very nimble to avoid unwanted uppercuts from flailing arms and fists. I recall one such incident very clearly—a huge sailor chap, obviously a heavy drinker, came in one day. Dr. Long called me to stand by—in case. The anesthetic was just under way, when the sailor yelled, "Turn on more steam," so I opened the cylinder of gas. A second shout from him again demanded more steam. Suddenly the strap broke. He was out of the chair; and what he did to our furniture had to be seen to be believed!

Equally suddenly, he stopped shouting and turning, looked about him and said, "What caused all the smashup?" Then he sat down in the chair and said "Take out that tooth." He refused a local and never moved a muscle while a difficult tooth was removed."

While the medical community ignored nitrous oxide, the public kept snorting and disporting, and Colton continued his exhibitions. In 1862, during a demonstration in New Britain, Connecticut, a woman asked Colton if he would give her nitrous oxide so that her dentist could extract one of her teeth. As he had almost twenty years before, Colton agreed, providing a bag of gas to Dr. Dunham, her dentist. As before, the operation was a success, transforming Dunham into an outspoken advocate of the anesthetic.

Dunham proved to be a much more effective prostheletizer than Wells, and within a year, with gas supplied by Colton, had administered it successfully to more than 600 patients. "It took the whole city by fire," according to one account. "People rushed in great number and had their teeth extracted, not only without pain, but in the inebriated state of exhilaration brought on by the gas." From the middle of 1863 through the following February, one New Haven dentist, Dr. Joseph H. Smith, extracted no less than 3,929 teeth with nitrous oxide— 1,785 in one month according to another account.

Colton, the itinerant lecturer had finally seen the future and it wasn't in public demonstrations. He went to New York and set up the Colton Dental Association on 22 Bond Street, working with several leading dentists. In less than a decade the Colton Dental Association, with branches across the United States specializing in tooth extractions, announced that nitrous oxide had been administered successfully on its premises over 27,000 times.

Meanwhile, Dr. S. Coult, aka Samuel Colt, who'd made audiences swoon as a teen with his gas demonstrations, switched from working with a product that killed pain to one that just plain killed, earning fame and fortune as the designer of the world's first mass-produced revolver. Indeed, it was the profits from his nitrous oxide demonstrations that allowed him to continue research and development of his handgun.

John Riggs, who had performed the extraction on Horace Wells, became Dr. Riggs, now known as the father of periodontal disease.

Wells himself, though he would ultimately earn posterity's gratitude, would come to a miserable end, as we will see in the story of ether. W. T. G. Morton, Wells's former student would also play a part in this numbing tragedy.

Ether—A Knockout Advance

ETHER WAS FINALLY receiving attention for its analgesic properties, showcased the same way laughing gas was demonstrated to the public. Georgia practitioner Dr. Crawford Long, a later claimant for the title of anesthesia's discoverer, recalled first noticing ether's painkilling power at such "ether frolics."

> On numerous occasions I inhaled ether for its exhilarating properties, and would frequently, at some short time subsequent to its inhalation, discover bruised or painful spots on my person which I had no recollection of causing, and which I felt satisfied were received whilst under the influence of ether. I noticed my friends while etherised received falls and blows which I believed were sufficient to produce pain on a person not in a state of anaesthesia, and on questioning them they uniformly assured me that they did not feel the least pain from these accidents.

Long's claim to the discovery of anesthesia arises from accounts of his having used ether during minor operations beginning in 1842. But he failed to report his experiences until 1848. The first documented use of ether as an anesthetic occurred in 1846, when one Eban Frost came to W. T. G. Morton, Wells's former student, for an extraction, asking if he could be Mesmerized to avoid pain. Morton told him he "had something better." Morton saturated a handkerchief with sulfuric ether, knocked the patient out, and removed a firmly rooted bicuspid. The grateful Frost wrote a testimonial testifying to the miracle.

> This is to certify, that I applied to Dr. Morton at six o'clock this evening, September 30th, 1846, suffering under the most violent toothache; that Dr. Morton took out his pocket handkerchief, saturated with a preparation of his, from which I

breathed from about half a minute, and then was lost in sleep.
In an instant more I woke and saw my tooth lying on the floor.
I did not experience the slightest pain whatever. I remained
twenty minutes in his office afterwards, and felt no unpleasant
effects from the operation

Eban Frost

An account was carried in the next days Boston's *Daily Journal*:

Last evening, as we were informed by gentlemen who witnessed
the operation, an ulcerated tooth was extracted from the mouth
of an individual without giving him the slightest pain. He was
put into a kind of sleep, by inhaling a preparation, the effects
of which lasted for about three-quarters of a minute, just long
enough to extract the tooth.

Morton soon had a thriving practice in painless toothpulling. But
where had he learned the secret of ether? According to accounts, the
suggestion came from Charles Thomas Jackson, a distinguished physician and surgeon with whom Morton had taken up practice. Jackson
had recommended Morton use ether to alleviate a toothache of his own.
A few drops proved efficacious, and Morton soon was experimenting
with ether, first on family dog Nig, then on goldfish.

The day after the painless extraction, Morton filed a joint patent
with Jackson, claiming to "have invented or discovered a new and
useful improvement in surgical operations on animals." The reference
to animals was reportedly due to Jackson's concern about possible
censure from the Massachusetts Medical Society, were it known they
tested their new invention on humans. Within two months, Morton
formed a dental partnership with Nathan C. Keep to exploit the commercial possibilities of the new anesthetic. Public notice appeared in
the *Evening Traveller*:

The subscribers having associated themselves in the business
of dental surgery, would respectfully invite their friends to call
on them at their rooms, No. 19 Tremont Row. They confidently
believe that the increased facilities which their united experience will afford them of performing operations with elegance
and dispatch, and the additional advantage of having them per-

formed without pain by the use of the fluid recently invented by Doctors Jackson and Morton, will not only meet the wishes of their former patients, but secure to them additional patronage.

Yet Morton sought ever greater recognition and respect for himself and the discovery he now claimed almost total credit for. He sought to arrange a demonstration of ether at the Massachusetts General Hospital, similar to the exhibition Wells had attempted. But as Morton refused to identify the ingredients of his invention, the medical society refused to let the demonstration take place. Finally Morton relented, and on October 16, 1846, Dr. John C. Warren—who'd also overseen Wells's disastrous demonstration—used ether to anesthetize a patient and painlessly remove a tumor from the man's neck. "Gentlemen," the professor announced to the class in the operating theater at the conclusion of the operation, "this is no humbug." Morton received United States patent #4848 for his invention, which he called "letheon," that same month.

Reaction in the medical society was immediate. In the minutes of the meeting following the operation, the record shows members were incensed at the "scandal" and determined to stop further such exhibitions. "We cannot allow Professor Warren, in his credulity, and out of the kindness of his heart, to become a tool of a vicious little dentist," they wrote.

Others recognized the advance for the landmark it was. Oliver Wendell Holmes, poet, physician, and father of the later Supreme Court chief justice of the same name, was moved to overheat his prose past the boiling point as he sought to articulate the meaning of the miracle:

Nature herself is working out the primal curse which doomed the tenderest of her creatures to the sharpest of her trials, but the fierce extremity of suffering has been steeped in the waters of forgetfulness, and the deepest furrow in the knotted brow of agony has been smoothed for ever.

What to call the state of consciousness, or the lack of it, that the ether induced? It was called the "sleeping-gas operation," the substance called simply the "mixture," "preparation," "gas," "new discovery," or Morton's fluid. Morton and his circle promoted the name "letheon," taken from the river Lethe of Greek mythology. The myth held that a draught of the water of Lethe could "expunge all painful memories," as Holmes wrote. Holmes, a professor of anatomy at Harvard, entered the fray himself in a letter to Morton in November of 1846:

> Dear Sir,
> Everybody wants to have a hand in a great discovery. All I do is to give you a hint or two, as to names, or the name, to be applied to the state produced and agent. The state should, I think be called "Anaesthesia," The objective will be "Anaesthetic." Thus we might say "the state of anaesthesia," or "the anaesthetic state." I would have a name pretty soon, and consult some accomplished scholar, such as President Everett or Bigelow, Senior before fixing upon terms which will be repeated by the tongue of every civilized race of mankind.
> Respectfully yours,
> Oliver Wendell Holmes.

Based on this letter, Holmes has been given credit in some quarters with coining the term, but the word anesthesia first appeared in English in the *Dictionary Britannicum* in 1721, predating its use in connection with the application of ether by more than 120 years.

When news of the Morton's discovery reached England in mid-December it was received with much excitement. Two days later, a London dentist used ether during the extraction of a molar. Surgeons used it in an operation at University College Hospital two days later.

The $100,000 Question

FOLLOWING MORTON'S SUCCESS and coronation as the discoverer of anesthesia, Wells came forward to claim credit for his place in history. He first experimented with nitrous oxide, hadn't he? He'd given up his molar in the name of science! Indeed, he'd even worked with Morton, introducing him to the properties of anesthetic gas. But Wells's claims were rejected at Boston General Hospital and everywhere else.

This was more than a matter of honor. With the surgical suffering wrought by the Civil War, Congress had posted a $100,000 prize to the inventor of anesthesia, whomever it might be. Morton's recognition for the discovery of the application of anesthetics in surgical use had put him on the inside track to claim the prize. He even succeeded in prevailing on Congress to up his award to $200,000, citing its value to the army and navy. But more claimants arose, and before Morton could be paid, each claim had to be thoroughly investigated.

Meanwhile Wells, dejected but determined to spread the gospel of anesthetics, set out for New York intending to introduce nitrous oxide to hospitals and dentists. But a new drug craze was sweeping the nascent anesthetic world: Chloroform. It had been independently discovered in the early 1830s in the United States, France, and Germany and introduced as general anesthesia in 1847 by Dr. James Young Simpson, who published a lengthy report on its superiority over ether.

Wells acquired a couple of gallons and began experimenting. Without patients, there was only one subject available. As told in one account, "Day after day he slumbered under the influence of chloroform vapour, and the result was inevitable—he became a chloroform addict . . . chloroform became indispensable to him."

It was not long before Wells was seen as a vagrant tramp, roaming the dark streets of New York. The only companions he could find were the prostitutes of the city, the beggars and the drunkards of the obscure underworld. Soon even these began to shun him which, of course, made matters worse. Horace Wells was toppling head over heels into the realm of madness. One day, believing the whole world was against him, particularly the despicable outcasts and prostitutes, Wells bought a bottle of vitriol and threw it upon two girls who happened to pass by. Amidst the screams of pain and agony, a great multitude assembled, and it was a wonder that Wells was not lynched there and then; the police managed to rescue him with great effort.

Following a speedy court appearance, Wells was remanded to prison. He explained his assault on the women thus in a letter: "coming out of a stupor and exhilarated beyond measure," he told of seizing a vial of acid from the mantel, rushing into the street, and hurling the contents at a pair of prostitutes plying their trade there.

He lasted only a few days behind bars. On the morning of January 24, 1848, a guard looking through the spy hole on the cell door noted Wells "crumpled into a peculiar position." Horace Wells was dead at age thirty-three. The elixir with which he sought to end the world's suffering now eased the last of his. Somehow he'd managed to conceal chloroform on his person or acquire it while incarcerated. After taking a large dose, he'd severed a femoral artery in his thigh and bled to death.

Wells's martyrdom fueled the flames of the controversy surrounding credit for the invention of anesthesia. Morton's enemies blamed him for Wells's suicide and the battle between their camps embroiled all manner of believers and apologists on each side. Then another claimant for the honor—and the cash—appeared: Professor Jackson, Morton's ex-partner.

According to Jackson, he'd identified ether's anesthetic properties in 1842, after knocking over a jar with chlorine gas he was preparing, first nearly suffocating and then suffering from a terrible sore throat. The next day, he said, he inhaled ether vapor to reduce the throat discomfort, was thrown into a state of insensibility, and realized he could use ether to deaden pain.

Morton, he said, came to see him on September 30, 1846, the date that Eban Frost received his painless extraction. According to Jackson, it was at that meeting that he told Morton about the anesthetic properties of ether, of which his visitor had been totally ignorant.

Though Jackson was regarded, superficially at least, as a respectable professional, a routine background investigation would have revealed decay on the X-ray of his soul. (Not that Morton didn't have skeletons in his closet, or somewhere. He brought a skeleton, that on his honeymoon, and on their wedding night his bride awoke alone in bed and, searching for her groom, discovered him alone with the skeleton.)

Most telling of Jackson's character was his involvement in a dispute with Samuel Morse, inventor of the telegraph. The two had met on an ocean crossing in 1839. After Morse patented and published his invention, the electromagnetic telegraph, to great acclaim two years later, Jackson claimed the invention was his. He said Morse stole the idea during their ocean voyage. Jackson's efforts to win credit for the invention were especially nettlesome to Morse in Europe.

During subsequent court proceedings, Morse described Jackson as a "lunatic" and "intolerable nuisance." It took Morse "seven years and half his wealth to clear his name and get the well-deserved priority of being the inventor of the telegraph."

Jackson was not so successful in his claim for inventing anesthesia. Soon realizing the campaign was doomed, he instead set about trying to sabotage Morton's stake in the honor, enlisting Wells's widow and a senator in his effort. After finding an article in the *Medical Journal of Georgia* about an old slave who'd had two fingers amputated painlessly by Dr. Crawford Long in 1842, Jackson traveled south, found the ex-slave as well as Dr. Long and interviewed them both.

Meanwhile, dentist Dr. John F. Brewster Flagg, son of early American dentist Josiah Flagg, exposed Morton's "new compound letheon" as nothing more than washed sulfuric ether combined with aromatics to disguise its odor. Therefore it could not be patented.

Congress, fed up with the competing claims for the cash awaiting the anointed discover of anesthesia, finally withdrew the prize altogether. Meanwhile, the rapid and widespread use of ether resulted in several deaths, even when administered under proper conditions. Charges about Morton's efforts to claim total credit for its discovery led many to regard ether and Morton both as a menace. Many dentists who used ether refused to use the inhaling apparatus Morton invented for its use. Ultimately, Morton's dental practice was ruined, and he became the object of ongoing attacks from the health community.

Morton died destitute in 1868, at the age of forty-nine. Still Jackson continued trying to ruin his reputation, his efforts escalating from campaign to obsession. On a sunny day in July, 1873, Jackson was strolling through a park in Boston, headed in the direction of Mount Auburn Cemetery. According to a contemporary account, a beautiful shining monument he passed caught his eye. Jackson stopped long enough to read the inscription:

WILLIAM T. G. MORTON

INVENTOR AND REVEALER OF ANESTHETIC INHALATION
BY WHOM PAIN IN SURGERY WAS ANNULLED;
BEFORE WHOM IN ALL TIME SURGERY WAS AGONY,
SINCE WHOM SCIENCE HAS CONTROL OF PAIN.

ERECTED BY THE CITIZENS OF BOSTON

Jackson "uttered a piercing cry and flung himself onto the statue, trying with his fingers to tear it to pieces. Soon an assembly gathered round, staring at the unusual sight of the raving maniac." An ambulance arrived and Dr. Jackson was taken to the McLean Asylum for Lunatics in Somerville. He lived out his days there, lasting another dozen years before dying in 1880.

Wells ultimately received posthumous recognition for his seminal work in the development of anesthetics. In 1864 the American Dental Association gave full credit to Dr. Wells. In 1870 the American Medical Association followed suit, resolving that he discovered practical anesthesia. A monument to him was erected in Hartford's Bushnell Park, and on the fiftieth anniversary of that first anesthetized extraction, a bronze bust of Wells was installed in the Army Medical Museum in Washington, DC.

Wells's widow was hardly mollified by his posthumous honors. She said his discovery, a priceless gift that paved the way for our nerve-deadened epoch of painless dentistry "had been to her and her family and unspeakable evil," for it cost the life of her husband.

6

Licensed to Drill

Dentistry in the Era of Robber Barons and
Reformers

T HE NINETEENTH CENTURY WAS AN ERA OF GRAND AMBITIONS
and nefarious schemes, of progressive reformers, unscrupulous
con artists, and greedy tycoons. All these trends and trendsetters,
symptomatic of the young nation's teething pains, were represented
within dentistry. A struggle for the soul of the evolving profession,
between America's twin promises of unfettered freedom and uniform
justice, was underway, waged in the wide-open spaces of its citizens'
mouths.

Professionals Put Down Roots

As THE EIGHTEENTH century drew to a close, the skilled itinerant dentist was getting tired feet. He began to abandon his migratory ways,
establishing himself in one location. Soon all the top practitioners of
the day were operating from a permanent address. Without the need to
update prospective patients on their whereabouts, respected dentists
began to turn away from using newspaper advertisements to promote
their services. Soon, the road circuit and the newspaper ads became
the sole province of the "itinerant empiric," or "floater."

Dentist Benjamin James warned of the dangers of dealing with
these fly-by-night road warriors in *Treatise on the Management of the
Teeth*, published in 1814.

> Most people maybe deceived at the time of an operation; though
> woeful experience in a few months unfolds the deception. The
> impostor is sought for to make reparation, or to receive merited

punishment; but the bird has flown; he is gone to practice his tricks and deceptions among those, who know not his character; until prudence drives him into another seclusion from revenge, into another 'shoal of dudgeons.'

In all occupations, it is safer to employ those only, whose permanent residence enables us, at all times, to call them into account for negligence or deception. The itinerant dentist ought, therefore, never to be trusted.

Empirical Evidence

CONCERNS ABOUT QUACKS and empirics became topic numero uno among dentists seeking acceptance as a professional class. And with good reason. Governance of the trade was virtually nonexistent. Even an educated consumer had trouble identifying the uneducated quack. Early in 1800s anyone could buy a dental degree for five to twenty dollars from diploma mills like the Central University of Medicine and Science of Jersey City or the Philadelphia University of Medicine and Surgery. Complaints regarding the widespread lack of professional training and warnings against charlatans were recurring themes in dental literature of the era. B. T. Longbothom's *A Treatise On Dentistry*, published in 1802, was among the first:

> The word Dentist, has been so infamously abused by ignorant pretenders, and is in general so indifferently understood, that I cannot forbear giving what I conceive to be its original meaning,

His book spelled out the services he felt a qualified dentist of the day should provide, which included "cleaning, extracting, replacing by transplantation and making artificial teeth." This was in sharp contrast to the public's limited perception of dental duties, according to charges he leveled in an ad in *The Federal Gazette and Baltimore Advertiser* that same year:

> The tooth-drawing mechanic and the barber-dentist has fatally erected a standard whereby the ignorant form their notions, and unthinkingly annex to tooth-drawing and toothscraping all that is requisite to be known.

American dental literature had been born in the century's inaugural year, 1801, with the publication of R. C. Skinner's "A Treatise on the Human Teeth." The sixty-eight-page work combined basic information on dental care and hygiene with claims for Skinner's own superiority in his field. For the next half-century, tracts such as this would become the sole method, besides hands-on practice, by which an education in dentistry was acquired.

Leonard Koecker (1785–1850), who practiced in Baltimore, Philadelphia, and London, bemoaned the inevitable results of the lack of standards in *Principles of Surgery*:

This unsettled and vague state of practical Dental Surgery, not only exposes the profession and the unwary public to the errors of the dentist, but it also leaves the greatest opening for the most impudent and ignorant pretenders to assume a profession, which they utterly disgrace. . . . It is a well-known fact that there are quacks in every professions, and in every country; but it cannot be denied that they most particularly abound in the United States of America and England.

Noted dentist Levi Spear Parmly shifted the blame for the "slow progress of dental sciences" to society's lack of respect for the field. In *A Practical Guide to the Management of the Teeth* (1819), he griped that "the practice of it has generally been considered in no higher light than a mechanical occupation or trade."

The public's low opinion of dentistry was matched by that of fashionable physicians and surgeons. As one of the latter wrote in the English journal *The Forceps* in the 1840s, "A pure surgeon . . . can scarcely be expected to pay any attention to a subject of such minor importance as the teeth, or soil his aristocratic fingers by touching a key instrument."

Parmly's prescription for progress: "A great improvement of this department of surgery, will depend on pointing out to society the importance of preventing diseases of the teeth." Parmly vaguely suggested an institution for this kind of training and education, but nothing came of it.

Parmly's own interest in dental education had been sparked by the inspiring sight of mineral teeth in the mouth of a "French gentleman" in Pittsburgh, a beautiful gold filling he examined in New Orleans (done by distinguished London dentist George Waite), an impressive "swaged" gold plate, and other state-of-the-art Continental dental work he'd seen.

"Soon afterwards I embarked for London, with as full and strong a determination as I think was ever felt by a human being, never again to touch the shores of my native country, until I should know exactly how all these things were done."

After returning from two years in Europe in 1821, Parmly set up a practice in New York and became one of the era's most respected dentists.

Reform School

WITH A COUNTRY full of cavities and an absence of regulations, dentists proliferated. There had been about 100 dentists in the United States in 1825. The depression of the 1830s drove many unemployed mechanics to take up the practice, and in the two years after 1836, the number of American dentists nearly doubled. By 1840 the number had grown to 1,200.

In 1835 the *New York Mirror* noted, "We have often been struck with admiration at the vast increase in the number of dentists practicing in this city within the last few years; we can remember, and that not very long ago, when there were but six or eight, and at present, we are informed that the list is swelled to eighty."

What struck many other observers was not admiration. Noted one, "The calling of dentist seems to be considered open ground into which any fellow who has impudence, some steadiness of hand, and a case of instruments, thinks himself free to take up a position."

American dentist Shearjashub Spooner (1809–1859) was in the vanguard of those calling for reform. Born in Vermont, Shearjashub trained under his brother, John, in Montreal. In 1838 he sounded a clarion call to dentists to remove the decay from their midst.

One thing is certain, this profession must either rise or sink. If means are not taken to suppress and discountenance the malpractices of the multitude of incompetent persons, who are pressing into it, merely for the sake of its emolument, it must sink;—for the few competent and well-educated men, who are now upholding it, will abandon a disreputable profession, in a country of enterprise like ours, and turn their attention to some other calling more congenial to the feelings of honorable and enlightened men.

Spooner, a rabid foe of empirics, suggested how to root out and keep the decay from recurring: "The dental profession should be protected by legislative enactment; every person before he be permitted to practice it, should serve a term of pupillage and pass an examination before a competent board of dentists." Furthermore, "that means be taken to improve the mass of dentists throughout the country—*to purge the profession*" [original italics].

England was in equal need of regulation. A dentist at the Royal Free Hospital noted in 1850: "Falstaff, himself, never possessed a more heterogeneous, non-descript army than those who compose the majority of dentists in England. Having failed in every other department they consider themselves perfectly competent to practice as dentists. . . . The adage that any fool will do for a parson may be applied with still greater force and truth to the profession as a dentist."

Not all reputable practitioners were eager to end dentistry-as-usual. As respected a dentist as Eleazar Parmly, brother of Levi Spear Parmly, wrote, "Of all the distinguished men who have preceded us in our professional art, whose operations secured to them the greatest name, and to their patients the greatest good; there was no one among them, as far as I am acquainted with the history of dentists, who was at the outset of his professional career, 'medically educated.' "

Meanwhile Parmly, like many other leading dentists, was helping solve the education problem one student at a time. He charged $1,000 per student to teach dentist wannabes the trade.

Foil Rap

WHETHER A DENTIST was good or bad, a professional visit remained a nerve-wracking, or wrecking, prospect in preanesthesia days. The simple act of filling a cavity remained brutal and barbarous; little changed from the 1400s. The accepted method called for using hand instruments to laboriously dig away the decay, an excruciating process. To fill the tooth, gold foil was pounded into place, as painful a procedure as digging out the decay.

Dentists needed a filling material that was more malleable and less expensive than gold, one that was easy to prepare and apply, and impervious to the harsh chemical tides of salivation that washed over the teeth. Alternatives began to appear in the late 1700s, based on a combination, or amalgam, of mercury with one or more metals. The Chinese had used an amalgam of mercury and silver for filling teeth in the eleventh and twelfth centuries, but had themselves forgotten about it. In 1826, M. Taveau of Paris introduced such a "silver paste" to the West. Composed of filings of pure silver blended with mercury, this was the first modern amalgam.

There were drawbacks to early amalgams, most notably that mercury, the essential ingredient, is poisonous. Though rendered nontoxic when it bonds with other metals, the mercury in early amalgams did not completely combine with the other constituents. Many physicians of the era used calomel, or mercurous chloride, as an all-purpose remedy, and it was coming under increasing attack due to the dangers mercury posed to the system. Meanwhile, dentists were increasingly alarmed by the dangers of mercury in amalgam, and the majority of leading practitioners opposed its use.

An additional problem for amalgams was the temperature at which early versions needed to be applied. The first European formulations had to be poured into cavities at over 200 degrees. That was quite painful when contacting an exposed nerve. Also, the behavior of amalgam as it hardened was poorly understood. It could expand upon setting, or contract. Thus, depending on the shape of the cavity and the behavior of the amalgam as it solidified, the filling could shrink and fall out or enlarge and shatter the tooth.

Yet these early flaws were not the reasons the acceptance of amalgam was delayed for decades within the dental community. The delay was the result of the chicanery of amalgam's greatest promoters, the Crawcours, and their product, Royal Mineral Succedaneum.

A Royal Scandal

IN LATE 1820s and early 1830s French dentists working in Great Britain began advertising the latest amalgam for filling teeth: mineral succedaneum. Said to be the equal of gold for use as a filling material, its main competitive advantage was that a tooth could be filled with mineral succedaneum "in about two minutes without the slightest pain, inconvenience, or pressure."

Claiming to be "the sole and original proprietors" of this preparation were the Crawcours. But who were these dental magicians? In most advertisements they referred to themselves simply as Mr. or Messrs. Crawcour, so information on the number and names of individuals is impossible to ascertain. But as a family they have been described as "notorious empirics of Polish extraction." They appeared in France, where members acquired a rudimentary knowledge of dentistry, and soon were billing themselves as "surgeon-dentists." The first arrived in England by the late 1700s and was soon working the cities and towns in the country's north.

Their activity heated up in the 1800s. Amid a blaze of saturation advertising, the Crawcours "systematically visited innumerable cities and towns" across England filling teeth. In 1833 they prefixed "Royal" to their compound's name and elevated their own standing to surgeon-dentists to the Royal Family, patronized by the Courts of Austria, Belgium, France, Russia, and Prussia.

A subsequent analysis of Royal Succedaneum found it to be "an amalgam of mercury—poisonous in its quality, subject to rapid oxidation, and therefore, totally unfit for use, in the case of diseased teeth," mixed with coarse filings from French silver coins. Their amalgam was also prone to significant expansion upon hardening, resulting in many fractured teeth. As for the fast service, a Crawcour didn't bother removing decay and carious portions of a tooth before applying the amalgam, unless required to anchor the filling. In the wake of their ministrations, inflammation of tooth pulps (pulpitis) and abscesses of tooth sockets frequently followed.

In 1833 two of the Crawcour brothers descended on America. Described as "elegant and enterprising," they introduced the royal compound in New York with the same saturation-style campaign used to such good effect in Europe. Their ads spoke of "a few moments' reclining in a luxurious easy-chair," undergoing "the gentle insinuation" of the amalgam. The ease of the procedure made them hugely popular. In a matter of months they amassed a fortune and were treating the (former) top clientele of the city's best dentists.

Native dentists grew outraged—both at the practices of the Crawcours and their own loss of business. A backlash built, erupting into a long battle against the Crawcours and amalgam itself, a conflict that would become known as the Amalgam War (1835–1850).

The Amalgam War

HEALTH PROBLEMS SOON began cropping up among the Crawcours' patients. The high mercury content of their amalgam became known. Dentists spread the word on the dangers of mercurial salivation that often accompanied use of Royal Mineral Succedaneum. Shearjashub Spooner called the Crawcours "swindling villains." Eleazer Parmly, brother of Levi Parmly, developed an opposition to the pair that "amounted to an obsession" according to one account.

With Parmly's prodding, local dentists organized the Society of Surgeon Dentists of the City and State of New York. Officers of the Society posted a notice in *The US Medical and Surgical Journal* stating their mission to "promote the respectability of the profession, by putting down, if possible, all imposition and unprincipled quackery, by which the public and the profession at large are made to suffer." Every member of the society was required to sign a pledge never to use amalgam under any circumstances. Any who refused were expelled.

The campaign succeeded in arousing public ire, and by the end of 1834 the Crawcours had fled America. However, the Amalgam War had just begun. Though the enemy had retreated from the field of battle, amalgam remained. Many dentists regarded it as a dangerous weapon that had to be disarmed and banned. But its ease of use continued to make amalgam an attractive alternative to fillings-as-usual. And given the loud denunciations against it, one can infer there were more than just a few pockets of resistance.

Dentist Solyman Brown proclaimed in 1839 "that this execrable material is still used by some unprincipled men in this country."

Some would vouchsafe Brown's intimate familiarity with execrable material; he is known to cognoscenti of bad poetry for writing some of the most dreadful verse executed in English, grand epics dedicated to dental subjects. In works such as "Dentologia: a Poem on the Disease of the Teeth and Their Proper Remedies" and "Dental Hygeia, a Poem on the Health and Preservation of the Teeth," Brown demonstrated that whatever pain he inflicted on the teeth was more than matched by paeans he inflicted on the ears.

In 1839, the American Society of Dental Surgeons was formed in response to the amalgam controversy. Its stated mission was "to promote union and harmony among all respectable and well-informed dental surgeons, to advance the science by free communication and interchange of sentiments either written or verbal, between the members of the society both in this and in other countries, to give character and respectability to the profession by establishing a line of distinction between the truly meritorious and skillful and such as riot in ill-gotten fruit of unblushing impudence and empiricism." Despite the even-handed language of the charter, the society was a front organization for amalgam opponents, and worked ardently to further its anti-amalgam agenda.

The war raged on the frontier, as well. Ohio's established dentists went on the attack against the cut-rate itinerant empirics. The Mississippi Valley Association declared its contempt for amalgam fillings in 1844, an action taken, as one member said, "from a desire on the part of every member present to separate ourselves so far as possible in faith and practice, from a certain class of operators who made a free and reprehensible use of amalgam."

In 1846, the American Society of Dental Surgeons passed a resolution compelling every member to sign a pledge not to use amalgam under any circumstances, and avowing that its use constituted malpractice. Vigilante teams were formed to spy on members and assure they were in compliance. Several dentists were expelled, others resigned.

The Society of Surgeon Dentists of the City and State of New York had already been shuttered by similar internal warfare. Parmly's rabid antipathy toward amalgam had caused disputes that led "to the final destruction of the Society." Now the same fate was befalling the dental surgeons. The casualties were taking too high a toll on the profession. After years of warfare, dentists had seen enough bloodshed.

In 1850, the American Society of Dental Surgeons rescinded its amalgam resolution. The Amalgam War was over. But peace was uneasy. Though improved alloys were introduced, like one from Elisha Townsend of Philadelphia in 1855, amalgam continued to be scorned by many dentists. Quality varied between batches and was not always prepared the same way. Silver, the major ingredient in these amalgams, came from United States coins. One bad batch of amalgam was attributed to having been made with silver from Mexican dollars. A good, workable amalgam was finally developed in 1895 by America's "grand old man in dentistry," G. V. (Greene Vardiman) Black (1836–1915), paving the way for universal acceptance of amalgam.

Nowadays amalgam fillings have progressed considerably from the Crawcours' time. In the comforting words of modern dental texts, the mercury in contemporary compounds "generally becomes nontoxic to most individuals in its amalgam form."

Meanwhile, back in Europe, the Crawcours dropped Royal Mineral Succedaneum in favor of an entirely new filling material they claimed to have discovered: Royal Asiatic Puzzolano. Their advertisements reported the improvement speeded up the procedure so the filling "is performed in a few seconds, inserted in a soft state without pain or pressure, hardens into enamel, allays the most excruciating pain, prevents the necessity of extraction and lasts for years."

Later analysis showed it to be identical to Royal Mineral Succedeneum.

Drill Instructors

THE FIGHT AGAINST the Crawcours and the attacks on empirics and charlatans was part of a larger effort aimed at bringing accreditation and regulation to the profession, presaging the reform movements that would later sweep many social, business, and government institutions. The longer action was delayed, the greater the signs a thorough cleaning was needed.

Among the loudest voices for educational reform belonged to esteemed dentists Chapin A. Harris and Horace Hayden. Harris authored America's first professional dental book, *The Dental Art: a Practical Treatise on Dental Surgery*, published in 1839. This has been labeled the "birth year of organized dentistry" in some quarters, for the number of firsts it witnessed. In addition to Harris's book, the charter for the world's first dental college, the Baltimore College of Dental Surgery, was granted, which Harris and Hayden founded. Additionally the first dental journal, *American Journal of Dental Science*—edited by Harris—appeared. And in one more landmark event, the aforementioned

American Society of Dental Surgeons, a pioneering organization, was established.

Of all these events, the founding of the Baltimore College of Dental Surgery, the world's first dental college, which opened in 1840, was by far the most revolutionary. It ushered in the era of formal dental education and the development of modern dental techniques and training that would make the United States the world leader in dentistry.

The dental business was booming, the growing commerce and commercialism reflected in the ever larger number and variety of dental instruments. Traditional small dental cases were no longer sufficient to hold them. Soon wooden boxes were being jerry-rigged into service, outfitted to hold all the tools of the trade. John D. Chevalier invented what is considered the first practical dental instrument case, a five-compartment model that gained wide popularity among mid-century dentists. To simplify one-stop shopping for this and other products, Chevalier opened the world's first dental supply house in 1833 in New York. By 1840 Chevalier was creating exquisite, bejeweled dental instruments that were works of art as well as superb, albeit unsanitary, tools.

The first commercially manufactured dental chairs became available in about 1850, thanks to the merging of dentistry and industry engineered by Samuel Stockton White. In 1844 he opened the S. S. White Dental Mfg. Co., the world's first dental manufacturing company, in Philadelphia. S. S. White became to dentists what Sears, Roebuck and Co. would become to rural America. Beginning with tooth molds and expanding to instruments and furniture after the Civil War, the company remained in the forefront of dental supplies worldwide well into the twentieth century.

White wanted his company to be a source of information as well as supplies. Beginning in 1847, the company published the *Dental News Letter*, continuing as the *Dental Cosmos*, a well-known journal of the era, in 1859. White's literary legacy survives today, the result of *Cosmos*'s merger with the *Journal of the American Dental Association* (*JADA*) in 1936. Today the *JADA* remains the preeminent publication of American dentistry. White was also instrumental in the long legal battle over the patents on vulcanite dentures, a tale of monopoly, greed, and death, which will be examined in the following chapter.

The Rank and the File

SOON AFTER MID-CENTURY, the Baltimore College of Dental Surgery and a handful of other dental schools were turning out qualified dentists. But these grads could hardly meet the needs of the populace, and there was still nothing to stop anyone who wanted from filling the gap. In the absence of government oversight, reputable dentists argued for an organization by which to sanction and regulate their members. Earlier efforts at unification, such as those inspired by the amalgam controversy, had ended in failure. A group of twenty-six like-minded dentists gathered at Niagara Falls in 1859 to act upon that goal.

The resulting professional body, born if not conceived at the honeymoon haven, was the American Dental Association (ADA), which would become the primary voice of the country's dental establishment. One of the first issues addressed was the undignified practice of advertising. The ADA Code of Ethics, adopted in 1866, banned advertising and personal solicitation.

In the aftermath of the Civil War, dentists in the south seceded from the ADA, banding together in the Southern Dental Association (SDA), formed in Atlanta in 1869. The SDA remerged with the ADA in 1897, becoming the National Dental Association, before the association's name was restored to the original in 1922. The advertising prohibition enacted in 1866 remained in effect until 1977.

States, meanwhile, prodded by organized dentists, passed their own laws regulating dentistry, the first enacted by New York in 1868. By the early 1900s, all states had dental-practice acts of varying degrees of strictness. California and many western states had rather loose regulations.

State dental societies passed their own restrictions, too. The Dental Society of the State of New York's code, adopted in 1868, proclaimed: "In order to more effectively promote the honor of the profession, as well as to preserve good feeling and learning among its members, it shall not be deemed honorable for any member, by means of advertisements, handbills, circulators, or in conversations with his patients, to claim to be the exclusive manufacturer or possessor of good incorruptible or other teeth; or to claim any superiority over any other member, either as to his mode of performing any operation or the quality or kind of teeth, or other material or instrument used by him."

Of course, professional societies' ethics code were only enforceable on members of the society, which wasn't a requirement for the practice of dentistry.

The Civil War–Armed to the Teeth

WAR BRINGS OUT the best and worst in man, and in the Civil War, the same might be said for dentistry. Some men avoided service to their country through acts of dental self-mutilation. Conscripts needed two or more opposing front teeth to qualify for induction; these teeth were essential in ripping open the paper envelopes containing gunpowder. Several objectors had their front teeth extracted prior to the induction examinations, rendering themselves unfit for duty.

On the positive side, the longer-ranged rifles, higher-caliber armaments, and more effective shrapnel led to a significant increase in wounds involving the head and face. These injuries accounted for about 10 percent of all battlefield casualties, and the demand this created for oral surgeons helped the field to make bold advances during the war years. The Confederacy appears to be the clear victor in this theater of operations, having established wards in at least three hospitals devoted to maxillofacial surgery.

Following the war, dental departments were gradually established in hospitals across the country, a trend that continued to the turn of the century.

Grant's Tomb and Grant's Tooth

PARADOXICALLY, ONE OF the most intriguing episodes at the nexus of the Civil War and civil dentistry occurred long after hostilities formally ceased. The incident leads one to pose a question: could ex-President Ulysses S. Grant, former commander of the Union Army, have been assassinated by a Confederate spy—his dentist? The answer is undoubtedly no, but from the standards of modern conspiracy theorists, circumstantial evidence to the contrary is intriguing to say the least.

The facts of the case were brought to light by dental historian Dr. John Hyson Jr., director of curatorial services at the Dr. Samuel D. Harris National Museum of Dentistry in Baltimore, located on the site of the world's first dental college.

General Grant's death from cancer on July 23, 1885, has been attributed by many to a disease of dental origin. It was theorized that a broken molar was the initial source of the irritation at the base of the tongue which, aggravated by smoking, turned cancerous, soon involving the pharynx and lymph glands. Yet the background of one of the dentists treating Grant when the flawed repair set the disease process in motion was not fully investigated at the time of death.

Dr. Henry A. Parr was New York's top dentist. A graduate of the Baltimore College of Dental Surgery, the nation's finest, he reportedly enjoyed the highest income of any dentist in the city. But a simple background security check would have raised flags regarding the fashionable doctor. That he was a graduate of the class of 1884, and thus had presumably been practicing without a degree, was of little concern. Many dentists of the era practiced without accreditation. More problematic was his career as a high-level Confederate secret agent and spy during the Civil War.

Dr. Parr has been called "obviously . . . a confederate to the end." A known contributor of Confederate veterans groups, among his personal artifacts was a lock of Jefferson Davis's hair. One must wonder what went through the former operative's mind when General Grant, the ex-leader of the Union forces, now under his command, opened wide.

Parr's origins are vague. He was born in either Nova Scotia, New York, or Tennessee sometime around 1843. At the outbreak of the war he was living in Tennessee, and joined up with the infamous Morgan's Raiders, led my General John Hunt Morgan's Second Kentucky Cavalry. The date of his switch to the shadowy world of espionage is unknown, but by 1864 he was being paid from a special fund earmarked for clandestine activities controlled by Confederate President Jefferson Davis himself. In the midst of the war, he went under deep cover for the Confederate secret service, working as a drugstore clerk in Nashville. He teamed up with a man the Northern press called the "notorious Lieutenant Braine" in 1863, and together they engineered a series of hijackings on the high seas. They seized the Union steamship *Chesapeake*, the side-wheeler *Roanoke*, and a third ship that became the

Confederate's last raider afloat in the Caribbean.

The war's conclusion found Parr in Yarmouth, Canada, where he put his wartime training to use. He took a job in a drugstore, and became a pharmacist. By the time of his 1869 marriage, he listed his occupation as "druggist" and was later recognized as one of Yarmouth county's "pioneer" pharmacists. He was recognized in the United States as something else: a terrorist.

Confidential sources told United States federal agents that Parr would arrive in the country in June of 1878. He was arrested and charged with murder for the death of the Chesapeake's engineer during the "piratical seizure" of the ship. The case went to trial but the charges were finally dropped. It was proved Parr held a commission under the Confederate government, and was therefore covered by the presidential proclamation of amnesty.

Parr returned to Canada and gradually began practicing medicine as well as selling drugs, becoming known by the honorific "Dr. Parr." Following a fire that destroyed his pharmacy (he was insured for $5,000), he moved to New York and began practicing medicine full-time.

At what point treatment of Grant's molar began is unknown. While Parr was not his primary dentist, and indeed was not even involved in treating the troublesome tooth, his notorious past went unremarked following the general's death. If there was any talk at the time of either a conspiracy or a lone dentist theory, it was kept out of the press. The general went to Grant's Tomb and the doctor went on to invent devices such as his antiseptic telephone mouthpiece attachment. ("It purifies, protects the nose and throat." "Like your toothbrush used only by you.")

Yet the Teflon dentist did not stay out of jail forever. He wound up behind bars—albeit very briefly—in the aftermath of what became known as the "trial of the century," the case of the murder of architect Stanford White. Among Parr's star patients was Harry K. Thaw, the accused murderer. The incarcerated Thaw needed dental care, and Dr. Parr attended to him in his cell in the Tombs in 1906.

In an interesting coda that perhaps presaged the black-bag jobs of the Watergate era, an unknown person or persons broke into Dr. Parr's office on New York's Forty-second street in 1926, gained access to the safe, and stole President Grant's, Mrs. Grant's, and President Chester Arthur's dentures.

Leeching on Patients

DESPITE ADVANCES IN commerce, equipment, and education, dentistry retained some of its atavistic practices. Bleeding was still a staple of dental prophylaxis, recommended for relief of irritated gums and sundry other oral problems. If a standard procedure went awry, an extraction, for example, leaving a patient in discomfort or distress, bleeding might be recommended. The medical literature of the era contains numerous cases of patients who withered and passed on despite such ceaseless efforts to save them. In other words, they were bled to death.

Leeches were also a standard dental treatment of the era. *Systems of Dental Surgery,* published in 1835 advised, "Leeches on the gums over inflamed teeth often have a happy effect. If the incisors or canine teeth are inflamed and tender, a few leeches will alleviate all pain and tenderness in a very short time. With proper prudence on the part of the patient, and a faithful performance of the foregoing directions, inflammation of any of the teeth, or their membranes and nerves, or of the lining membranes of these sockets will very rarely take place."

It was hoped that patients responded well to the leeching, for if they exhibited a "disordered state" during these treatments, the book advised resorting to "Heroic Therapy," a comprehensive combination of bleeding, purging, vomiting, and blistering a patient until his condition showed signs of improvement.

Leeches were applied in dentistry into the twentieth century. Their use was well described in 1917 by Charles Edmund Kells, a dental pioneer of his own age. Kells still used them, for example in cases of pericementitis, the progressive necrosis of the alveolus, or tooth socket. They were kept in stock by druggists even in Kells's day. He reported "it is rare indeed that it is not possible to obtain one when it is needed." His leeches were imported, the best coming from the Dalmatian coast, shipped in hundred-leech lots in small wooden tubs packed with their native soil.

Kells highly recommended their use to dentists. "To all who meet with occasional periodontal troubles after filling root canals or, in fact, any other conditions involving local inflammation, leeches are really invaluable and all such should feel they are not doing their full duty to their patients unless they use this means of relief," he wrote.

However, from his comments we can see leeching was an art in itself. They were not the most compliant creatures. First the leech needed to be coaxed or corralled into a "leech tube," something like an oversized eyedropper without the rubber stopper. The end of the tube was then placed over the afflicted area of the gum, thus directing the leech to its workplace. Kells described this process as "tedious." It could take twenty to thirty minutes—and was fraught with unanticipated perils.

"Sometimes a lively little fellow will be coming out of the little end of the tube before it can be placed on the gum. In that case, withdraw the tube quickly, for if he starts going down the patient's throat, said patient may manifest a slight doubt as to one's being a real leech artist."

Applying the leech to the proper spot was no guarantee of success, either: "There is an old saying that you can drive a mule into the water up to his ears, but you cannot make him drink, and so it is with the leech."

Even if the leech's compliance was secured, leeching was no easy procedure to endure: "Once the leech starts sucking blood, it must not be disturbed and so patient and operator must remain absolutely still."

And one final caveat: "A leech should never be used a second time."

Equal Opportunity Openings

WOMEN AND MINORITIES of the age also found opportunities in the burgeoning profession—initially, at least. Colonial records reveal a black dentist, Peter Hawkins of Richmond, Virginia, was practicing as early as 1765. He was said to be "a tall, raw-boned, very black Negro, who rode a raw-boned black horse, for his practice was too extensive to be managed on foot, and he carried all his instruments, consisting of two or three pullikins, in his pocket. His dexterity was such that he has been known to be stopped in the street by one of his distressed brethren . . . and to relieve him of the offending tooth, gratuitously, without dismounting from his horse. His strength of wrist was such, that he would almost infallibly extract, or break a tooth, whether the right or wrong one."

In South Carolina a slave, Cesar, was freed in 1792 after rendering dental and medical "cures," and given an annuity of $100 by the state assembly.

By 1840 about 10 percent of the 1,200 dentists in America were black. Blacks needed their own dentists because white dentists often refused to treat them—even though some of the most noted dentists of the day employed blacks as assistants.

A black, Robert T. Freeman, was in the first class of six graduates from the Harvard Dental School in 1869. The Howard University College of Dentistry, founded in 1881 provided another training ground for minority dentists. Yet growth of black dentists stalled, then declined. By 1910 there were more than 30,000 dentists in the United States, yet less than 500—not even 2 percent—were black.

Women also struggled to enter the field. Emeline Roberts Jones was among the first. After marrying a dentist in 1854, she tried to get him to teach her the trade. No dice. Women didn't have the constitution or dexterity needed, he told her. Emaline decided to teach herself. She began making off with extracted teeth from his office and practiced filling them at home in secret. Only after having drilled and filled hundreds this way did she reveal her handiwork to her husband. Obviously impressed with her work, he took her on as a professional partner. Following his death a decade later, she carried on the practice alone for half a century, earning the honor as America's first female dentist.

Lucy Hobbs Taylor faced similar obstacles on her way to becoming the first woman in the United States to receive a dental degree, in 1866. Even after training as an apprentice dentist, she was turned down for admission to the Ohio College of Dental Surgery twice, strictly due to her gender, before the school finally accepted her.

Many Eastern schools were even more reluctant to accept women than Ohio College had been. In 1868, James Truman, a professor at the Pennsylvania College of Dentistry mounted a vigorous campaign to have women admitted to dental schools, identifying his own institution as one that henceforth would. Subsequent changes in admission policies brought more women to the field, and by 1880 there were more than 600 women practicing dentistry in the United States. In 1890 Ida Gray became the first black woman to earn a DDS degree, bestowed by the University of Michigan School of Dentistry. However, for women as for blacks, troop strength within the civilian dental corps was declining. By the year of Gray's graduation, the number of women dentists in the United States had fallen to some 330.

Though academicians of the time may have been resistant to the idea of women dentists, potential patients were not. After the Ohio College of Dental Surgery undertook an effort to bring more women into dentistry, the *Cincinnati Dental Reporter* editorialized thusly:

> We heartily second [the school's efforts]. Even now we almost imagine ourselves seated in what is usually termed the "chair of Torture"—dreaded now no more—by our side a beautiful lady, with sweet breath and glowing cheek, her delicate arm encircling our head, our cheek resting against a busom still more soft, looking up into her eyes, so tender in their gaze— they take away all dread, and in their sympathy even divide the pain itself. With such a dentist, we would want our teeth examined every twenty-four hours.

Attitudes toward women dentists as expressed in the foregoing, may help explain the decline in their ranks following their early gains. A poem published in England's *Punch* in 1887, "To a Lady Dentist," reveals such sentiments were not confined to America.

> *Lady Dentist, dear thou art,*
> *Thou has stolen all my heart;*
> *Take two, I shall not repine,*
> *Modest molars such as mine;*
> *Draw them out at thine own sweet will,*
> *Pain can come not from thy skill.*

> *Lady Dentist, hear me pray,*
> *Thou wilt visit me each day;*
> *Welcome is the hand that comes—*
> *Lightly hovering o're my gums.*
> *Not a throne, love, could compare*
> *With thine operating chair.*

Lady dentist, fair to see
Are the forceps held by thee;
Lest those pretty lips should pout,
You may pull my eye teeth out;
I'm regardless of the pangs
When thy hand extracts the fangs.

Lady Dentist, when in sooth
You've extracted every tooth,
Take me toothless to thine arms,
For the future will have charms;
Artificial teeth shall be
Work for you and joy for me.

The Era of American Dentistry

IN A MATTER of decades the young nation had transformed itself into a dental superpower. American dentists seized global attention at the first world's fair, London's Exhibition of Industry of All Nations, in 1851, taking top honors in dentistry with their displays of artificial teeth, crowns, bridgework and regulation (straightening) of teeth. By 1870 there were 13,000 members of organized dentistry. Average annual income was about $1,460. The country boasted nine dental colleges. None existed in Europe or Asia. So-called "American dentistry" became a designation used worldwide, signifying advanced practices and procedures. Many of these American-style practitioners had no claim to anything American other than possibly speaking a word or two of English. One Swiss dentist, for example, was educated in Germany, trained in France, spoke no English, yet hung out a sign advertising "American Dentist" in Cairo, Egypt. But some were actual expatriates. One such American in Paris would amass a fortune while helping influence the fate of Europe, thanks to his unique ability to combine dentistry and diplomacy.

Thomas Evans arrived in Paris fresh from winning an award for his gold fillings at Philadelphia's Franklin Institute in 1847, after just four years in practice. The award earned him a position with a top American dentist already practicing in the City of Light and Evans quickly became a favorite of the upper-crust clientele. Appointed by Napoléon

III as "Surgeon-Dentist" to the imperial court, Evans was soon sought after by royalty across Europe, not only for his dentistry, but as a trusted conduit for information among heads of state, bypassing normal diplomatic channels. He attended to royalty in Holland, Germany, Austria, Belgium, and Russia.

In Paris he confidentially—and confidently—warned Americans of the impending Franco-Prussian War two weeks before its outbreak. Setbacks in the conflict roused a Parisian mob to storm the palace, demanding the blood of the Napoléon III's wife, Empress Eúgenie. It was Evans who whisked her to safety, a clandestine escape and 100-mile odyssey recounted in a true-life adventure-thriller, *The Dentist and the Empress.*

Evans far outlasted his original royal benefactor and became a fixture on the international social circuit. He never charged his important patients for dental work, either, instead using the inside information they gave him to grow rich investing in real estate. He was worth $4–10 million at the time of his death. Much of his wealth and the priceless treasures he'd acquired as gifts from grateful patients and potentates became the basis of Philadelphia's Thomas W. Evans Museum and Institute. What little remains today is under the stewardship of the University of Pennsylvania, most of the Evans's collection having been subsequently sold or auctioned.

The Tooth of a Literary Lion

AS DENTISTRY BECAME identified as an American specialty, it was only natural that the most American of storytellers, Mark Twain, would take an interest in its tale.

Before sailing to Europe at the start of a round-the-world lecture tour, Twain was said to have heard the story of the first use of laughing gas in dentistry directly from Dr. Riggs, the man who performed the initial painless extraction. Desirous of hearing the story again, Twain engaged Dr. Riggs to overhaul his teeth. He got the story, but he also got a bill for $200 for the two days of work, reportedly bringing a frown to the noted humorist. Wrote a contemporary:

They say Twain was so mad that he didn't get over it till the seasickness incident on the passage of the Atlantic worked the bile out of his system. He has not yet offered Dr. Riggs's story for publication. Neither has he paid the doctor's bill.

One can advance two plausible reasons for the nonpayment. First, Twain might have been feeling the effects of the financial ruin he suffered when his publishing company went bankrupt. Second, perhaps the work hadn't been completed to his satisfaction. In a subsequent account of his travels in England, Twain recalled a toothache he experienced in London, the pain triggering Proustian recollections of the dentists' office back home.

One night that tooth did jump, and every time it jumped it raised my head right off the pillow. How I did lie awake and think about that dentist's shop in Elmira, where I had been under torture so many times—of those pretty dental instruments, so polished and so cold! How I did long to lay my cheek against one—one of those short, thick, heavy twisted chaps, with the bow-legged, fluted and curved handles, and short haws-bill jaws! How I reveled in delight at the thought of having such a thing clutch my refractory tooth and "yank it!" With what pleasurable emotions came crowding into my mind the recollections of that dentist and his room and his fixtures—his big easy chair, with the pretty white-curtained window before it, and the nice, big, red glass spittoon to the left, with the hole in the bottom, and the bits of red cotton and the bright pieces of gold and streams of blood-stained saliva on the sides. And then, the pretty little bureau with the bottles on the top and the little yellow drawers which he jerks out so gently when seeking for some new and more delicate instrument of torture. And then that beautiful little round, velvet-covered stand on the gas fixture in front, covered with the nice drills, and pretty files, and the lovely little crowbars with the stained ivory handles, and the long steel crochet needles with which he hunts for new cavities, and the little round pasteboard box full of gold "plugs" and the dirty little napkin and the rubber ball syringe, and the singular smell of his thumb, and all that! Oh, how nice.

Twain's may be considered the minority voice in his celebration of the implements of dentistry. A more commonly held attitude toward the tools of the trade and those who wielded them was expressed by a writer for the *Chicago Herald*:

> His instruments of torture, called by courtesy dental tools, were many and varied. He was very skillful in his profession and when he took a job he did it in first-class style. The dental tools are simply copies in miniature of articles used in the Spanish inquisition and on refractory prisoners in the Tower of London. There are monkey wrenches, raspers, files, gouges, cleavers, pickes, squeezers, drills, daggers, little crowbars, punches, chisels, pincers and long wire feelers with prehensile, palpitating tips, that can reach down through the roots of a throbbing tooth and fish up a yell from your inner consciousness. When a painstaking dentist cannot hurt you with the cold steel, he lights a small alcohol lamp and heats one of his little spades red hot, and hovers over you with an expectant smile.
>
> Then he deftly inserts this into your mouth and when you give a yell he says, "Does that hurt?"

Parlor Games

THE LATE NINETEENTH century witnessed the rapid spread of dental parlors and unrelenting dental advertising. The "painless" dental rooms, or "parlors" had appeared as early as the 1830s, advertised by crude trading cards, such as one for a Dr. Manson in Brooklyn, spotlighting his use of "benumbing Gasoline, (no pain or danger)." As these rooms and parlors began to proliferate, regional chains spread. No licenses were needed to open, no training required to operate on patients. It was the unfettered expression of a free-market economy without government intervention. Yet it failed to deliver the greatest good to the greatest number of people. Bait-and-switch tactics, low-paid staffs, and inferior service were hallmarks of their operations. The extractions these parlors specialized in were not performed on patients' teeth, either, as explained in one account:

> The most important and best-paid job was that of the contractor. He was the diagnostician and the super salesman. To qualify for this all-important job he had to possess a pleasing, dignified

personality, be a good dentist and a student of human nature, particularly its weaknesses. The diagnosis was important, but only secondary to probing the depths of a patient's pockets.

In the eyes of the dental establishment, the worst of these practices and practitioners, the cheating parlors and their gaudy, undignified advertising, the incompetent itinerant and stationary scam artist, were personified by one of the best-known Americans of the age, now all but forgotten: Edgar Randolph Painless Parker. His story exemplifies the crosscurrents and evolution of turn-of-the-century dentistry, and documents the life of one of its most extraordinary and successful figures. It is examined at fascinating length in a biography subtitled, *A Dental Renegade's Fight to Make Advertising "Ethical,"* by Peter Pronych and Arden Christen.

Painless Parker

SHOWMAN, INNOVATOR, PUBLIC-HEALTH promoter, industry gadfly, and mogul of the mouth, Parker was born in New Brunswick, Canada, in 1872. At age seventeen, after a youth spent working as a peddler and seaman, he thought about his future and considered becoming a physician.

"It seemed to me," he recalled, "that all the doctors did was to stroll around in white coats, with great dignity and look cool. It didn't appear that they had to work very hard. They just looked scholarly and mysterious and prescribed sales. It looked like a good life, I knew I could look as mysterious and all-knowing as the next guy if I had one of those white coats on."

His mother, a devout Christian Scientist, was aghast, and Edgar dutifully reconsidered, and sought career guidance from a phrenologist. In the 1800s, phrenology (the pseudoscience of discerning one's character and temperament by analyzing the bumps on the cranium) was given the same level of respect that psychiatry (the analysis of bumps taken *within* the cranium) enjoys today. The phrenologist's evaluation, according to Dr. Parker:

His chart shows that he is outstanding along the mechanical lines and that he cares about people's health. He rates well up in other lines, too: the scientific, commercial and professional. However, in the final analysis, it all points to one thing—*he would make a good dentist.*

In 1889, Parker enrolled in the New York College of Dentistry and was soon working his way through college. "While the other boys were out studying, I was out getting enough to eat, via door-to-door dentistry. I carried my tools with me. I'd put my foot in a door and give a spiel patterned after the one I gave as a peddler. If I sold some dentistry, I'd start with the cook's teeth. If I didn't kill the cook, and was lucky, I'd eventually wind up working on the teeth of the lady of the house."

The approach had its limits.

"At first I would encounter problems that I hadn't yet come to in my dental-school education. So I'd have to come back later, when we reached the part of the course dealing with that problem."

After Parker's moonlighting got him expelled from college, he returned to New Brunswick and worked as an itinerant dentist, earning enough to enroll in the Philadelphia Dental College and Hospital of Oral Surgery (now Temple University School of Dentistry). Armed with a degree and its imprimatur of respectability, Parker gave up his itinerant ways and opened a proper dental office in New Brunswick. In three months he made seventy-five cents. Parker was at a crossroads. Would he continue to observe the rules of "ethical" dentistry, eschew advertising, and starve, or use the skills he'd learned as a peddler and his natural flair as a showman and huckster to make a success of his business?

"Why did I become 'unethical?,' " he later wrote. "Why did I leave the fold, break with regular dentists, go to practicing dentistry in my own chosen way, and face certain hatred and persistent persecution from the 'ethical' gentlemen? Well, hunger was the beginning—just a plain empty stomach that chattered louder than all the arguments and abuse of the dental colleges and dental associations in America."

Using the Salvation Army, Kickapoo Indian Medicine Company traveling medicine show, and his preacher's hellfire and brimstone diatribes as his inspiration, Parker wrote a sermon on the evils of oral-care neglect and set off to test it in a nearby town. After delivering the lecture he pitched extractions at fifty cents per tooth. He promised five dollars to any patient who felt any pain, a pledge Parker could offer due to his new painkilling discovery, "hydrocaine." Success was instantaneous.

"They needed dentistry worse than I needed money, if such a thing was possible . . . I took 33 teeth out of 12 patients and nobody screamed. Why, I'll never know; I ran out of hydrocaine on the seventh patient."

Painless Parker was born. In two weeks he was taking in as much as $50 a day. He traveled throughout the United States and Canada. Often, his efforts to practice were blocked by laws established by state and provincial dental authorities to regulate competition. He was busted on his twenty-first birthday for practicing without a license in Victoria, Canada.

He made it as far as Alaska, returned to the Maritime Provinces where he toured with his own vaudeville-style performing troupes, then moved to New York City. He established a thriving practice thanks to his tireless self-promotion and heavy advertising. Still, he periodically endeavored to "go straight" and hew to the strictures of the "ethical" dentists. That changed after he turned his career over to William Beebe, P. T. Barnum's former publicity agent.

Using a copy of *The Autobiography of P. T. Barnum* as his guide-book, Beebe designed saturation advertising campaigns and publicity stunts to make Painless Parker a household name. Soon Parker's building on Flatbush Avenue in Brooklyn sported huge signs on its sides. One read, "I am Positively IT in Painless Dentistry—Yes, Me! Painless Parker!" ("IT" was ten feet high.) The sign on the front of the building read:

PAINLESS PARKER,
PREEMINENT, PAR EXCELLENT, POSITIVELY PAINLESS
PERFECTION OF PRACTICE AND
PHILANTHROPICALLY PREDISPOSED TO POPULAR PRICES!

Performers of all types were engaged to parade before the building to drum up business. A tightrope walker in pink tights strolled on a cable in front of his edifice. He opened more clinics, hired more dentists. Billboards, magazines, newspapers, sandwich boards, walls of abandoned buildings, and almost every other conceivable formerly blank space now advertised his parlors. Crowds flocked. As for critics' complaints about the quality of dental care his clinics delivered, he offered a later rebuttal: "Regardless of what the ethicals used to say about us, the materials and workmanship of what we produced was OK."

Parker also took medicine shows on the road with troupes of thespians, singers, acrobats, jugglers, magicians, musicians, and tap dancers. Sometimes more than two dozen performers took part in these extravaganzas. A parade would precede the troupe's entrance into a town, with Painless Parker riding in a topcoat in an open carriage, sometimes throwing handfuls of nickels and dimes into the crowd. The climax of the shows was Parker's exhibition of painless tooth extractions. His principle anesthetics at these performances were said to be noise and confusion. Audience members were invited to seek his services at temporary quarters he'd arranged in their towns.

Parker became the butt of vaudeville jokes, and was labeled a "dentist gone bad" by New York's King's County Dental Society. He reveled in the notoriety, parading about with a seven-and-a-half carat diamond ring on his right and a four-and-a-half carat diamond tie stud. Like the tooth-drawers of old, he sometimes wore a necklace of teeth he'd pulled. It had 357 teeth—all extracted in one day.

In 1906 he left Brooklyn for California, planning, at age thirty-four, to retire. He brought with him somewhere between half and several million dollars, six railroad box cars of household furnishings, seven racehorses, and a new Model 15 Peerless Motor Car, the world's finest. But retirement and Parker proved a poor fit. Soon he'd bought a rundown dental practice in a bad part of Los Angeles and was back in business. (Parker liked sites "halfway between a slum and a luxury building.") Where in New York he used billboards and "human flies" crawling up walls to attract attention, in California he used blimps and banner-towing airplanes. He was a bigger thorn in the side of ethical dentists than ever—and more famous, as well. Hit with a barrage of lawsuits for fraud and malpractice, he responded aggressively and claimed he never paid out a penny in damages. The more he was attacked, the more he railed against the "Dental Trust," the malevolent forces of dentistry-as-usual that sought to restrain his exhibitions and activities.

Yet periodically he was still seized by impulses to go straight, and would temporarily give up his public demonstrations. Ultimately his hunger for contact with the crowd would become too great. He'd buy another vehicle, slap a dental platform onto it, hit the streets, and start his pitch again. But even that wasn't enough anymore. In 1913 he bought a circus. Now animals and acrobats jumped through hoops to ballyhoo the grand openings of his new offices.

The dental trust stepped up its attacks, bringing in politicians as allies. The California legislature passed a law in 1915 compelling dentists to practice under their legal names, a statute aimed directly at Painless Parker. Parker had his first name legally changed to Painless four months later.

Though the ethicals continued harassing Parker through the 1920s and into '30s, his tireless advocacy of oral health care for the masses ultimately brought him a measure of acceptance, if not respect. Six weeks after his death in 1952, the California State Dental Board ordered all advertising signs be removed from his offices. Almost overnight the name Painless Parker, once ubiquitous, disappeared from the American cityscape. The offices of his chains were sold to individual operators. The agony this prophet of painlessness caused so many in his chosen profession was over.

A Sequah to the Story

TURN-OF-THE-CENTURY ENGLAND WAS even a more wide-open dental landscape than America. Barbers still performed tooth extractions and dentistry was still unregulated. Its lawlessness suggested something of the frontier of the American West, a spirit manifest in the person of England's most celebrated practitioner of the dental and medical arts of the era: Sequah.

From the late 1880s to 1909, Sequah held England in his thrall. He staged an elaborate medicine show based on a mythic re-creation of the American West, a Buffalo Bill rip-off, if you will. His entourage included cowboys and Indians in feathered headdresses. Touring throughout the British Isles, he performed from atop a colossal, golden horse-drawn carriage.

Who was Sequah? The first was William Henry Hartley (1875–1924). British born, tall and sallow, in his stage persona he adapted the swaggering gait, dress, and accent of an American cowboy. The climax of the show was Sequah's performance of tooth extractions. While a brass band played, Sequah proclaimed himself capable of removing as many as eight teeth a minute, and quickly set about proving it. The blare of the band achieved its primary function, drowning out the cries emanating from the stage. But the heady atmosphere created by the music, the crowd, and the attainment of a turn-of-the-century version of fifteen minutes of fame may have been enough to overcome any sensation of pain. One commentator summed up the allure succinctly:

> . . . the novelty of having your teeth drawn with a trombone playing near your right ear, a big drum beating near your left, and the eyes of the crowd following every contortion of your features has an attraction in it almost irresistible.

With the crowd fired up from his amazing display, Sequah's own medicines and those of other more reputable but equally worthless concoctions were brought out for sale, like his "amazing" Prairie Flower medicine. It would probably sell equally well today, given its ecologically and politically correct formulation. It was derived, he claimed, from concoctions of the Apaches and other American tribes, made from herbs from Montana and Dakota, and roots and mineral water from the far west.

Hartley ultimately retired from his self-created role, but Sequah went on. So popular was he and so sophisticated the marketing machine behind the larger-than-life figure of the hard-riding, tooth-wrangling tough guy, that eventually there were twenty or more Sequahs, operated under the direction of the Sequah Limited Organization. Fittingly, the successor company finally came under the control of an American, John Morgan Richards, who added popular American quack remedies to the stock of products. Soon Brits were enjoying the imagined benefits of Carter's Little Liver Pills, Dr. Williams Pink Pills for Pale People, and Antikamnia Tonic. Finally, the last Sequahs rode off into the sunset when the Sequah Medicine Company Limited was dissolved on March 26, 1909.

7

False Promise

Dentures and Dental Prosthetics through History

O F ALL MANUFACTURED GOODS, PERHAPS ONLY THE TOUPEE IS the butt of more jokes than the denture. Even their accepted name, false teeth, brands them as dishonorable, outcasts in the oral cavity they would make their home. All the denture cleansers in the world are not sufficient to erase the stain of ridicule heaped upon them. How unjust that this device, a holy grail for centuries of prosthetic artisans and edentulous dreamers, should be held up to scorn. Perhaps the tide will turn. As society embraces more that is false, from values to a growing array of new and remodeled body parts, we are sure to develop a genuine appreciation for these artificial wonders.

Bridging the Gap

THE SEARCH FOR suitable replacement teeth has doubtless been going on as long as originals have been absent. Finding teeth was easy enough—ones already fallen out, animal teeth, dead people's teeth— but how to hold them in place, make them functional, and enable them to stand up to the massive vertical and lateral pressures generated by the masticating jaw?

The dental bridges left by the Etruscans and Romans mark the beginning of the answer to the problem. The engineering minimiracles they constructed have been discussed. Yet even then, some saw in dentures a reflection of society's own artifice. The first-century Roman poet and satirist Martial (Marcus Valerius Martialis) mocked them in his verse. To a contemporary woman of style, Gall, he taunted, "You are arrayed in the height of fashion and your tresses are manufactured far away, and you lay aside your teeth at night just as you do your silk dresses."

He gave another denture-wearing lady of privilege a stronger tooth lashing: "You use, and are not ashamed, teeth and hair that you have bought. What will you do for an eye, Laelia? That cannot be bought."

Martial might have been pleased that after the fall of the Roman Empire, dental prosthetic arts went into retrograde. The crude replacement teeth fashioned during the Dark Ages marked a nadir in dentistry's artificial intelligence. It was not for want of need. Loss of teeth could be health-threatening (aside from the danger one faced in the extraction process), owing to their role in eating. Food selection was limited and almost everything had to be chewed. But the tooth-drawers and barber-surgeons of the day specialized in taking teeth out, not putting them back in. Abulcasis, the Arab surgeon of the eleventh and twelfth centuries, suggested using bone to fill the gaps left by missing teeth. Two centuries later, European practitioners could apparently offer little better; Guy de Chauliac, the French surgeon who wrote with such surprising sophistication on other dental matters, was virtually silent on the subject.

Artificial Intelligence

THE RENAISSANCE SHAPED the development of dentures as it influenced the treatment of teeth. The flexible molds developed to take impressions of carvings, statuettes, and other decorative work for reproductions would later be adapted for denture-making. The molds allowed impressions of patients' gums and remaining teeth to be taken, so dentures could be designed for proper fit. Early molds weren't accurate enough for dental application, but since the recipe for the casting compound called for a witches brew of glue and ingredients including urine, perhaps it was just as well.

The teeth weren't the only part of the mouth to get restorative attention. In the 1500s, an artificial tongue tip was fashioned at the suggestion of the battle-tested French surgeon Ambroise Paré. Replacing a large section of a soldier's lost lingua, the disk-shaped piece of hardwood, hollowed on one side, slipped over the tongue's stump, and was attached to its owner with a string worn round the neck.

The earliest complete sets of dentures known (that is, full uppers and lowers), crude as they were, date from this same era. One pair was found in Japan, the other unearthed in Switzerland.

Dentures began to proliferate in the 1600s. Charles Allen's 1685 Book, *The Operator for the Teeth,* England's first book on dentistry, spoke enthusiastically of them:

> When our decay'd Teeth are so far gone before we think of any Remedy for their preservation, that whatever we do proves fruitless; and that notwithstanding all our best endeavors they . . . quite rot away, or that some intolerable pain has made us draw them: we are not yet to despair, and esteem ourselves Toothless for the rest of our Life; the loss indeed is great, but not irreparable, there is still some help for it; the natural want may be supplied artificially.

By end of the century artificial teeth were becoming common, as were the false promises of those selling them, as this ad from *The Ladies' Diary* of 1711 indicates:

> Artificial teeth set in so well as to eat with them, and not to be distinguish'd from natural, not to be taken out at night, as is by some falsely suggested, but may be worn for years together. They are an ornament to the mouth and greatly help the speech. Also, teeth clean'd and drawn, by John Watts (Operator) who applies himself wholly to the said business, and lives in Racquet Court, in Fleet Street, London.

Most early dentures were made from a variety of natural materials. The most common for the denture base was hippopotamus (called "sea horse") ivory. The teeth themselves were preferably human, though carved cow's teeth, elephant tusk, and walrus tusk were also used. Due to the action of saliva and other oral effluents, artificial teeth of bone and ivory began to darken and turn black within a year of use.

Whatever they looked like, they rarely felt right. Making the proper shape for an individual mouth was beyond the technology of the era. Practitioners simply outlined the jaw on a card or used a compass to take measurements of the mouth. From these crude approximations, the dimensions of the denture were obtained and the device carved. The resulting denture, so often promised to fit with perfect comfort over the gums, rarely fit at all.

A breakthrough in making a comfortable denture came from an unlikely place: Prussia, a land known more for square-jawed militarism than coddling the discomfited. In the mid-1700s, the technique of using wax to take an impression of a patient's teeth and gums was introduced. A plaster model was cast from the wax impression and became the template upon which dentures were made. Unfortunately, the advance was ignored by the dental world at large.

Partial dentures, which took the place of a limited number of missing teeth, were attached to neighboring teeth with thread or metallic ligatures, tied with the aid of fine-nosed pincers. This required a high degree of dexterity. Owing to the difficulty, once in place, the false teeth were usually kept there for extended periods, despite the discomfort their crude design caused. Being difficult to clean, the soon-stained partials resulted in a most cosmetically incorrect smile, "to say nothing," as one contemporary dentist said, "of this contaminating putrid accumulation being carried to the stomach of the unfortunate wearer."

Recycled Replacement Parts

THE PROVENANCE OF the human teeth used in these devices was questionable. During the eighteenth century, fabricators often assured clients they used "Waterloo teeth," that is, teeth harvested from soldiers who fell during Napoléon's final defeat. Battlefield scavengers routinely stripped corpses of teeth, for these were valuable commodities due to their use in dentures. Teeth of young soldiers struck down in the prime of life were apt to be vibrant and healthy, and at Waterloo, 50,000 corpses provided a bounteous harvest. The Peninsula War that raged between France and her opponents Spain, Portugal, and Great Britain in the Iberian peninsula from 1808 to 1814 was another source. Toothgatherers swept over the battlefields at the end of each engagement. Britain alone lost 36,000 men during the conflict. In the United States, tooth harvests were common in the aftermath of battles of the Civil War and Indian Wars. Teeth from dead Civil War soldiers were shipped to England by the barrelful.

Despite the supposedly copious supply of warriors' canines, cuspids, incisors, and molars, in reality, most of the teeth used in dentures were supplied by grave robbers, mortuaries, dissecting labs, and other places where riffraff, either living or dead, were likely to gather.

Body parts in general were difficult to come by. The need for cadavers for medical school dissection, when formal medical education was coming into vogue, was great. Government restrictions limited the supply available to anatomists in both the United States and Europe, heating up the market. By 1828, this was causing "fearful abuses" by "body snatchers." Grave robbers, called "resurrectionists," dug for their treasure, disinterring freshly buried bodies for their grisly trade.

Greed drove some to extremes. A pair of professional killers in Edinburgh, Scotland, William Burke and William Hare, sold their victims to the Edinburgh School of Anatomy, fetching ten pounds a cadaver. Sixteen bodies were sold, including a pair to the esteemed Professor Knox, a well-known lecturer in Old Surgeon's Hall. The professor claimed absolute ignorance of any untoward circumstances surrounding the acquisition of the specimens. Nonetheless he was subsequently "denounced by the clergy, hounded by the press, foully libeled and slandered, and physically attacked by the mob." The crowd that attacked him, described as "ribald," reportedly recited a quatrain during the assault on the once-esteemed professor:

> *Down the Clove and up the Stair*
> *But and ben wi' Burke and Hare,*
> *Burke's the butcher, Hare the thief;*
> *Knox the man that buys the beef!*

Upper Limits

ALTHOUGH FULL LOWER sets of teeth, held in place by gravity, were common, full uppers were rarely made. At least a pair of teeth was considered necessary for anchoring uppers in place. True to their heritage as fashion tastemakers, some Parisians without upper teeth submitted to having their gums pierced. From these stigmata, a set of dentures fitted with a pair of hooks could hang. This may have been acceptable for the avant-garde, but for most, no upper teeth translated into a life of undentured servitude. A force was needed to hold the uppers in place, and a mechanical solution was sought.

Early in the eighteenth century, whalebone strips were introduced, built into complete denture sets, pushing the upper and lower apart. Gradually the whalebone was supplanted by steel. Pierre Fauchard, the Father of Dentistry, developed the first effective method of attaching an upper set of teeth to a toothless jaw, using metal springs fixed to the lower set. The springs pushed the two halves apart. Then it was up to the gums and lips to keep the teeth where they belonged. Soon complete sets linked with spirals of silver and gold were seen in fashionable mouths. If only the uppers were needed, the spring could be attached to a frame that fit over a lower set of natural teeth.

Coils and springs had their drawbacks. They were hard to clean and difficult to master as recounted in *The Management of Artificial Teeth*, written by John Tomes in 1851:

> Teeth retained by spiral springs require considerable care in putting them in to the mouth. The wearer not infrequently injures or entirely destroys 2 or 3 pairs of springs by bad management, before experience has taught that manner of avoiding such accidents.

Even though uppers could now theoretically be held in place, making a workable set proved daunting. The standard horseshoe design of lower sets proved inherently unstable for uppers when subjected to real-world rigors of mouthwork. What was needed was a complete, proportioned denture that covered the entire palate. Hippo ivory was too difficult to carve into such a complex shape.

Thomas Berdmore, author of the landmark 1768 work, *Disorders and Deformities of the Teeth and Gums*, mentioned lack of stability among dentures' problems, even as he enumerated the benefits of artificial teeth:

> Although artificial Teeth are evidently ornamental; although they give a healthy juvenile air to the countenance, improve the tone of the voice, render pronunciation more agreeable and distinct, help mastication, and preserve the opposite Teeth from growing prominent; yet many are prejudiced against them on account of some inconveniences . . . they are said . . . not to sit easy on the gums:—Seldome to stand firm:—And to loosen after some time the neighbouring Teeth to which they are fas-

tened.—Or, the hard ligature, which is commonly used, is often
seen to cut very deep into sound Teeth.

Smooth Obturator

AMONG THE GREATEST contributing factors in advancing oral prosthetics was syphilis. It appeared in Naples in 1495, and remained a
scourge into the twentieth century. It claimed Henry VIII (in concert
with cirrhosis of the liver), in England, where a rumor in 1665 that
contracting syphilis warded off the plague sent men of London stream-
ing to the city's brothels. Symptoms of the venereally vectored epidemic
included destruction of the soft tissues and bones of the palate and
nose. This left a statistically significant segment of the population without a portion of the roof of their mouths, sometimes rendering them
speechless. A prosthetic remedy, an artificial palate was needed; in
contemporary parlance, an obturator. Amatus Lusitanus (1511–1561)
obliged the world by inventing the device. Plugs of metal, linen, and
sponge were among the early efforts of amelioration. Paré described
such an obturator.

> Sometimes a portion of the bone of the palate is destroyed by
> the shot of an arquebus, or some other wound or by a syphilitic
> ulcer, the patient being thereby disabled from properly pro-
> nouncing words and from making himself understood. To repair
> this defect we have found an expedient through the help and
> ministry of our art. It consists of the application of an instru-
> ment somewhat larger than the palatal perforation; this is made
> of gold or silver, of about the thickness of a crown (coin), and
> has the form of a vaulted roof to which a sponge is attached;
> when introduced into the aperture, the sponge, absorbing the
> humidity natural to such parts, will very soon swell up, and
> thus the instrument is held firm. In this way words are better
> pronounced.

The use of this style obturator was discontinued after it was discovered the swelling of the plugs, expanded by oozing pus from ulcerated tissue, accelerated tissue damage. Subsequent designs
incorporated ingenious solutions to hold the devices in place. One

artificial palate had butterfly wings which opened with a key once inserted in the sinus cavity. Others featured drainage holes for mucous.

The French Revolution

FRANCE OF THE 1700s remained unmindful of the denture-making advances on the Prussian front, displaying the same blissful ignorance that would have such tragic consequences in the Franco-Prussian War a century later. The French, however, sparked a revolution in dentures of their own with the introduction of "mineral teeth."

Dissatisfaction with the limitations of ivory led dentists to experiment with an advanced composite material: porcelain. A malleable paste of minerals, when fired, porcelain grew hard and strong. The development efforts resulted in the introduction of the one-piece "incorruptible" denture. To give the appearance of individual teeth, the one-piece dentures were painted. But early models were brittle, their color unnatural, and more important, the firing process shrank the porcelain, making it almost impossible to achieve the proper fit.

In the early 1770s, Alexis Duchâteau, a chemist from Saint-Germain-en-Laye, near Paris, was, like many, having troubles with his ivory dentures. Interested in porcelain teeth, he had a set made for himself at a china factory. Firing shrank the first set so much they were unwearable. Numerous others were made. When the size was right, the color wasn't—the porcelain initially made the teeth appear too white. When the color was rectified, the size was wrong again. Duchâteau began experimenting with a porcelain paste that vitrified (or fused) at a lower temperature. More failures followed.

In 1774, Duchâteau approached Parisian dentist Nicholas Dubois de Chémant and proposed working on the mineral teeth together. Modifying the paste, they finally producing a denture that fit Duchâteau reasonably well. Duchâteau attempted to market the product without success. For his efforts, Duchâteau received an accolade from the Royal Academy of Surgeons in Paris and nothing more. De Chémant, meanwhile, continued the experiments. He refined the paste, calculated the exact temperature for firing, and designed a spring system for the mineral teeth. In 1788 he published a book on his teeth and the following year King Louis XVI bestowed upon him an inventor's patent for mineral teeth. De Chémant announced his invention at the Academy of Science and Faculty of Medicine in Paris. It was a milestone in the history of dentistry, a technical breakthrough in the restorative arts, the first successful artificial teeth constructed entirely from inorganic material.

Soon, honors rained upon de Chémant. The Paris Faculty of Medicine declared that his dentures "united the qualities of beauty, solidity and comfort to the exigencies of hygiene." Edward Jenner, discoverer of the smallpox vaccination, gave de Chémant's product a celebrity testimonial, as did the President of the Royal Society of Medicine in Paris, Mssr. Geoffroy:

> I declare that the success is superior to my hopes. I further attest, that the teeth of sea horse which I wore for only one year, had so much disgusted me, by the bad smell they gave to my breath, and the disagreeable taste they communicated to my food, that I had not only withdrawn myself from company, but taken them out to eat.
>
> I no longer doubt, Sir, that my ill state of health proceeded from the putrid miasma given out by the bony substance of this set of teeth . . . since I have laid it aside, and have used yours, my health is infinitely improved. I eat with more facility . . .
>
> By your discovery, you have without doubt rendered a service to humanity; let us hope, that soon private gatherings and public places will no longer be infected by those animal substances . . . imagine two thousand people at the opera, there may be amongst them, at least, two or three hundred who have a small piece of sea horse tooth in the mouth; form an idea of all those decayed substances, and you will have a skeleton of the animal, which, if placed on the stage, would soon drive away all the spectators by the putrefaction and disgust it would occasion.

The elderly General Comte de Martagne was moved to wrote a poem in his honor:

> *When time has stripped our armoury bare,*
> *Dubois steps in with subtle heed;*
> *New grinders and new cutters gives;*
> *With his we laugh, with his we feed.*
> *Long live Chémant, friend in need.*

The accolades, along with de Chémant's claim of sole inventorship, inspired a backlash from other Parisian dentists and accusations that he didn't deserve full credit. Litigation was initiated at Duchâteau's insistence.

De Chémant ultimately established his legal right to the honor of inventor of mineral teeth. In 1792 he moved to London and won exclusive right to make dentures of porcelain paste for fourteen years. By 1804, he claimed some 12,000 of his dentures were in use. But the mania for one-piece porcelain dentures de Chémant provoked was finally ended by the incompetence of his imitators, who gave porcelain teeth a reputation for a poor, uncomfortable fit.

Terro-ist Tactics

THOUGH DE CHÉMANT'S mineral teeth failed to supplant those fashioned from natural substances, porcelain was by no means extracted from the future of artificial teeth. In 1809, single porcelain teeth were introduced by Fonzi, an Italian dentist practicing in Paris. He called them *dents à crampon*. Individually made, each tooth had a platinum stud soldered to a gold or platina base. Fonzi's porcelain teeth exhibited the subtle translucency of the genuine article.

Upon reaching England, news of the teeth set dental circles abuzz, as the following letter dispatched to a friend of the Fonz attests. The Ruspini it refers to was Bartholemew Ruspini.

Being at dinner the other day, with Chevalier Ruspini, Surgeon-Dentist to the Prince of Wales, and not a little occupied in masticating a fine haunch of roasted beef, teeth became the subject of conversation. Several kinds of artificial grinders were, of course, mentioned, and, among others, I took an opportunity to notice those with which your friend is now ornamenting the jaw bones of Parisians. This excited the curiosity of the Chevalier, who earnestly solicited me to assist him in getting a peep at his celebrated discovery; and brother Italian's late promising, that if he could approve of it, after examination, he would employ his utmost exertions to be of service to the author in England. He wished not only for a tooth or two, but to be informed of the manner in which they were fastened in."

Fonzi's teeth would be called "terro-metallic" in England. Non-decaying, their extended mouth life gave them a distinct advantage over other alternatives—including human teeth. But problems with lingual contour, dowel attachments, and base-bonding remained to be conquered. Ultimately these problems, along with their somewhat un-natural "bean shape" and the grating sound produced upon their meeting in the mouth, kept terro-metallic teeth confined to a cul de sac of dental history.

Still porcelain teeth would not die. They lived on in the far more refined "tube teeth" introduced by Claudius Ash of London of the late 1830s. These featured a central sleeve of gold or platinum which slipped over a post implanted in a denture base or tooth root.

The first porcelain teeth arrived in the United States in 1817 with Dr. A. A. Plantou, a French dentist, who introduced them in Philadelphia. As for the first full set of false teeth in America, the credit for their fitting is given to Robert Wooffendale, for the use of William Walton of New York. The set, as one dental journal later noted, "was thought to be a wonderful triumph of genius." Yet when it comes to denture firsts in America, the story must focus on the man who was first in war, first in peace, and can claim title, honorifically at least, as America's First denture wearer: George Washington, first president of the United States.

George Washington–The False Story

GEORGE WASHINGTON REMAINS one of the most recognizable Americans. His visage on the United States dollar bill, the stiff lips over which he stares back, help perpetuate a legend regarding Washington's "wooden" teeth. Washington's dentures were constructed of material typical of contemporaneous artificial teeth, including hippopotamus, walrus tusk, cow teeth, and elephant tusk. But not wood. Lead and what are thought to be elk teeth were used in one of his several sets of dentures. In the Gilbert Stuart portrait from which his countenance on our currency is adapted, Washington is wearing dentures with a hip-popotamus ivory base.

Yet there is nothing false about the portrait of Washington as a terminal toothache sufferer. As one writer put it, "Washington had the sort of teeth that decay fast and need prompt repair work." By the age of twenty-two, he began to lose teeth, and according to his meticulous accounts, expenditures for tooth extractions were made on an almost annual basis thereafter. He bought copious dental supplies and "spunge" toothbrushes by the dozens. A contemporary soldier describing Washington at age twenty-eight mentioned his bad teeth and reported he generally kept his mouth closed.

He began using partial dentures in his early forties and employed an army of oral-care specialists to help wage his campaign for oral tranquility. He enlisted the services of almost every well-known American dentist. John Greenwood, James Gardette, Charles Whitlock, and Jean Pierre Le Mayeur were among the commanders of the effort. It was a long, slow, and painful war of attrition.

Washington was said to suffer a recurrent toothache during the Revolutionary War. The outcome of the conflict and the coming out of his teeth exhibited interesting parallels. For both, the shortage of supplies and equipment was constant, the call for reinforcements and replacements unending. The desperate situation was reflected in his 1781 plea, dispatched to dentist John Baker in Philadelphia.

"A day or two ago I requested Col. Harrison to apply to you for a pair of Pincers to fasten the wire of my teeth.—I hope you furnished him with them.—I now wish you would send me one of your scrapers, as my teeth stand in need of cleaning, and I have little prospect of being in Philadelphia soon. It would come very safe by Post—and in return, the money shall be sent so soon as I have the cost of it."

Communication lines were not as secure as the general's intelligence apparatus led him to believe. The message was intercepted by the British and never reached Baker.

Most of Washington's dentures were not to his satisfaction. Yet uncomfortable and impractical as they were, he favored keeping them in during mealtimes. The resulting pain no doubt added to the "melancholy," a "certain anxiety," and "extreme sensibility" dinner guests commented on, and possibly contributed to the bouts of indigestion and short temper he was wont to exhibit.

Washington's last decade was capped by his 1789 installation as the first president of the United States of America. It would be a decade of dental discomfort that contributed to his declining health.

"At home all day—not well." "Still indisposed with an aching tooth, and swelled and inflamed gum," the president wrote in his diary on successive days in 1790. Ultimately, the only real tooth remaining in Washington's mouth was a lower premolar. By the time this last natural tooth was extracted in 1796, the dentures he was fitted with must have made chewing impossible. Instead of being anchored in place by teeth, his lips now took command of preventing the dentures' forward parry from his mouth. An English visitor in 1790 wrote, "His mouth was like no other I ever saw; the lips firm and the under jaw seemed to grasp the upper with force, as if the muscles were in full action when he sat still."

Perhaps the general was wearing that day the lead-base set combining human and the presumptive elk teeth, a denture with springs of coiled steel so powerful "that even today several strings of wire are needed to keep the upper and lower parts in contact."

The mental suffering this caused a man known as vain and concerned about appearances cannot be underestimated. Sensitive about the change in the shape of his face and his articulation, he reduced his public-speaking engagements.

Mrs. Washington fared little better. Left with a broken set of dentures in 1797, she gave them to Dr. Benjamin Fendall, who'd made them, for repair or replacement. A lengthy delay brought the general charging to the front lines of battle.

"Sir," he wrote to Fendall, "Mrs. Washington has been long in expectation of receiving what you took away unfinished, and was to have completed and sent to her:—and prays that it may be done without further delay, as she is in want of them and must apply elsewhere, if not done."

It may be comforting to those who consider poor service a modern development and anonymity its lubricant to learn the Father of his Country had to wait almost a year-and-a-half for this reply:

Dear Sir
    Within this Day, or two, I found myself, so much relieved, from my long continued and painfull illness, tho I use my left arm, with some difficulty, as to be enabled to finish Mrs. Washingtons [sic] Teeth, and you'll receive them, safe, I hope, by my Servant. They are nearly as I can now, recollect—like the old ones as there are so many ways, to make and shape Teeth— twou'd be almost impossible, to make them, exactly alike— after some time, without having the old ones present. The model, I took, has, also, by accident, sustained some injury. I

am extremely sorry, indeed, yr Lady has been obliged to wait so long—owing to my long absence from home and my Illness, after I had arrived at Cedar-Hill. I wish you and Mrs. Washington to have every conviction within yourself, I ever will with promptitude, and with pleasure, serve you both, whenever you may choose to command me—if in my power, and I fondly flatter myself, you'll both deem my excuse to be sufficiently admissible—at this Time. Please to present my most respectful comp. to Mrs. Washington & believe me, Dr. Sir.
Yrs with due respect,
B. Fendall

In the interim, Mrs. Washington had sought assistance from Charles Whitlock, in Boston, but busy with both stage performances and dentistry, he was unable to make a replacement set for her.

French-American dentist Le Mayeur, who specialized in tooth transplantation, treated Washington several times, staying overnight as a guest at Mt. Vernon. There is no record of him having done any transplants on Washington, but he transplanted five teeth for Washington's aide, Colonel Richard Varick. In a subsequent letter Washington wrote, "I have been staggered in my belief in the efficacy of transplantation of living teeth."

In what way he was staggered is not clear. However, twenty years after Le Mayeur's death, James Gardette wrote a follow-up report on transplants the dentist performed in Philadelphia. It was entitled "Observations on the Transplantation of Teeth, Which Tend to Show the Impossibility of the Success of that Operation." Gardette studied 170 cases, and "of these transplanted teeth not one succeeded," he said, though a few lasted a year.

Of all the president's dentists, John Greenwood was his favorite. Greenwood constructed three full sets and two partial sets of dentures for the general. In a letter of 1799, Washington advised him of his most-favored dentist status, and Greenwood used an extract from this communiqué in his subsequent advertising:

I shall always prefer your services to that of any other in the line of your present profession.

—George Washington.

Surely a ringing endorsement, coming from a man who could not tell a lie. That same year Washington's dental woes came to an end. He may have fallen victim to the standard treatment protocol of the day, according to an accusation made by a doctor against Washington's physicians shortly after his death.

". . . We see by their own statement," the accuser said of Drs. Craik and Dick, "that they drew from a man in the sixty-ninth year of his age, the enormous quantity of eighty-two ounces, or above two quarts and a half of blood in about thirteen hours. Very few of the most robust young men in the world could survive such a loss of blood; but the body of an aged person, must be so exhausted, and all his powers so weakened by it as to make his death speedy and inevitable."

Critics Bare Their Fangs

ADVANCES IN THE prosthetic arts were having an unintended affect. The closer false teeth came to their natural models and the more widespread their use, the more they were held up to scorn.

When they were exclusively for the rich in eighteenth-century England, no one thought to mock artificial teeth. They were no more real-looking then the fashionable piled wigs of the time, and weren't intended to appear natural or be functional. Diners typically took them out before coming to the table. Men returned them at the end of the meal to improve elocution over their after-dinner port.

The one-piece incorruptible denture, with its unnatural hue and the stiffness it brought to the countenance, was an early target of cartoonists and satirists. In the nineteenth century, the sense of shame associated with false teeth and the ridicule they drew rose in lockstep with advances in their construction. By 1840, artificial teeth, though cumbersome, had achieved an oddly lifelike appearance, which seemed to incite jokes and jibes. This reaction was partly in response to comical efforts owners took to hide their teeth's unnatural provenance, if not pretend they were real.

Scorn was directed not only at artificial teeth but users as well, of course. British prime minister Benjamin Disraeli blasted both at once in an attack on a rival Parliamentarian, saying his dentures "would fall out of his mouth when speaking if he did not hesitate and halt so in his talk."

The ubiquity of artificial teeth and changing attitudes about them is credited with affecting behavior in Britain during the Victorian age. The dry English wit of the period, it has been suggested, was developed so that gentlemen could avoid laughing out loud and showing their false teeth. The custom of eating in the bedroom prior to dinner that arose during the period has likewise been attributed to false teeth. After sating hunger upstairs without dentures, one could eat more demurely downstairs with them in place.

Yet for anyone of the era eager to snicker, many more were inclined to celebrate. Robert Rockliff established his position in the latter camp in "Address to A False Tooth," published in 1862.

> *They err who call thee false. Thou art, dear tooth,*
> *The very type of constancy and truth;*
> *For I have had thee long, and, since the day*
> *When first the dentist fixed thee in my jaw,*
> *Have found thee still impervious to decay,*
> *As perfect as a pearl without a flaw,*
> *An so exempt from every ache and pain*
> *From which my other teeth are seldom free,*
> *That I should reckon it no trifling tan*
> *Could I exchange the few that yet remain*
> *For sound and serviceable ones like thee.*

Yet as much joy as these devices brought to their owners, they could be unpleasant for others, as John Tomes reminded in *The Management of Artificial Teeth*:

It is of great importance that you should know how to preserve false teeth, for in the absence of proper attention they are soon destroyed, and still sooner become offensive. The wearer often seems singularly unconscious of the offensive odour which arises from neglected teeth—not so, however, the bystander; he is almost poisoned by the offensive breath of his neighbour . . . dentine [ivory], when highly polished, resists the action of the saliva, and therefore is not subject to decomposition. The wearer should pay great attention to this point. The surfaces of the teeth . . . should be well brushed with a little precipitated chalk, once or twice a day; and after brushing, rubbed with a dry soft towel.

Chewing Things Over

FOR THOSE WITHOUT teeth or dentures, masticators, which resembled large nutcrackers, could precrush and grind a mouthful-size portion of · food. Still in use at end of nineteenth century, they were sometimes recommended at the end of recipes in cookbooks of the day. An ad for one in a dental supplier's catalog of about 1880 explains the masticator's operation:

Invaluable to all persons with defective teeth
This instrument works on the principle of the action of the teeth. Meat and other food which requires masticating is easily and quickly prepared for digestion by the aid of the Masticator.

The food when ready for eating is first cut up into small pieces, which are then crushed with the Masticator into a pulp easily swallowed. The instrument is best worked if held almost horizontally with BOTH hands. To avoid chilling the food, dip the blades from time to time into hot water.

After use care must be taken to thoroughly cleanse the Masticator in hot water with a brush, and to rub it dry with a piece of chamois leather. It can be easily taken apart for the purpose of cleansing.

Artificial Teeth That Suck

PLATES COVERING THE whole roof of the mouth were barely considered before the 1830s due to technological limitations. Springs continued to be the force that kept uppers in place. James Gardette of Philadelphia made the first usable springless full palate uppers—unintentionally—in 1800, decades before their widespread acceptance. He carved a full upper for a woman and gave it to her to try out for fit before he'd put the springs on. Gardette's son, Emile, recounted what happened:

It was then still the custom for the dentists to attend at the houses of his patients, and a busy season caused months instead of weeks to elapse, when Mr. Gardette called again: with an apology for neglect, his pliers and springs ready, he requested Mrs. M'C. to bring the artificial pieces. She replied, "I have them in my mouth," much to the astonishment of her dentist . . . She stated that at first they were a little troublesome, but she had become accustomed to them now, and they answered every purpose as well without springs, and she was glad to dispense with them. The principle upon which the artificial piece thus adhered to the gums at once suggested itself to his mind, and suction, or atmospheric pressure, was henceforth depended upon in numbers cases of the same kind.

The later acceptance of plaster as a casting material, based on the Prussian model, led to the availability of the complete upper. The bases were often cast in gold. "Suction teeth," as they were called, were slower to catch on in England than in the United States, but by the 1860s and '70s they were all the rage, proclaimed as scientific marvels in advertisements, like one placed by Mr. G. H. Jones, Surgeon Dentist of London:

> Improved Prize Medal Teeth (London and Paris) are adapted in the most difficult and delicate cases, on a perfectly painless system, extraction of loose teeth or stumps being unnecessary, and by recent scientific discoveries and improvements in mechanical dentistry detection is rendered utterly impossible, both by close adjustment of the artificial teeth to the gums and their life-like appearance. By this patented invention complete mastication, extreme lightness, combined with strength and durability, are insured; useless bulk being obviated, articulation is rendered clear and distinct. In the administration of Nitrous Oxide Gas, Mr. G. H. JONES has introduced an entirely new process.

Dentures for the Masses—It Was a Very Goodyear

THE ADVENT OF anesthesia gave a terrific push to the demand for dentures. With extractions freed of pain, many more people rid themselves of rotted, aching teeth and sought artificial replacements. But before dentures could became mass-market merchandise, an alternative material, more malleable than ivory, less costly, and more comfortable than gold, was needed.

The answer was found on a house stove where ever-in-debt Charles Goodyear was experimenting with vulcanization—the process of turning raw rubber into a useful, pliable, and nonrotting material. He perfected the process in 1839 and received a patent in 1844. His brother Nelson figured out how to turn the soft, pliable substance to a hard rubber material he named Vulcanite, receiving a patent for it in 1851. A subsequent patent covering any resulting product as well as the manufacturing process was issued in 1858. By this time the Goodyears and companies licensed to make Vulcanite products were deep in patent infringement suits, suing process-poaching manufacturers. Daniel Webster was paid $25,000 in 1855, said to be the highest legal fee up to that time, to defend the patents in federal court on behalf of the company licensed to make Vulcanite shoes.

"I well remember that I had some experience in this matter myself," Webster told the court, in contrasting vulcanite with its predecessor and underscoring its unique properties. "A friend in New York sent me a very fine cloak of India rubber, and a hat of the same material. I did not succeed very well with them. I took the coat one day and set it out in the cold. It stood very well by itself. I surmounted it with the hat and many persons passing by supposed they saw standing by the porch the Farmer of Marshfield."

Meanwhile Vulcanite was being freely used by dentists in making denture bases. It ushered in what has been called "the era of false teeth for the masses" beginning in the 1850s. In 1848, Thomas W. Evans, the expatriate diplo-dentist, had used Vulcanite as a base for artificial teeth, and he made a Vulcanite denture for Goodyear himself in 1854. Vulcanite could be easily molded onto a replica of the patient's jaw, and the resulting base, once outfitted with porcelain teeth, would be perfectly fit, stable, didn't require springs, and was inexpensive. It was also a boon to those needing obturators, as Vulcanite allowed the devices to be fitted to the mouth more accurately than previous materials. It was hailed as the greatest advance in dentistry in a quarter century. The manufacturers of Vulcanite seemed content to let dentists use the material without paying licensing fees, and when Goodyear's original patent expired in 1861, dentists were convinced any threat of having to pay royalties on dentures had ended.

Not so fast. An obscure Boston dentist, John A. Cummings had been trying halfheartedly since 1852 to get a patent for dentures made with material Vulcanized by the Goodyear process. The patent office routinely rejected his applications. In 1864 he sent in another, with the exact same specifications and drawings previously submitted. Inexplicably, the patent was granted. Soon thereafter, Cummings transferred the rights to the Goodyear Dental Vulcanite Company. Noted dental historian Dr. Malvin Ring has uncovered many of the facts of this true-false test of the dental profession.

A Denture Monopoly

THE DRIVING FORCE behind the technology transfer was Josiah Bacon, an officer with the Goodyear Dental Company. Bacon soon had the company personally assign him ". . . the said letters-patent and all the rights thereby vested, together with the right to sue for and collect to his own use all damages for past infringements thereon." Bacon, it is surmised, had put Cummings up to reapply for the patent, figuring if it was successful and he could get the rights, a fortune was to be had.

With the rights in hand, Bacon demanded dentists obtain licenses. Dentists who wanted to use Vulcanite to make dentures would henceforth have to pay an annual fee to the company. Dentists were assessed fees of $25 to $100 per year, based on the size of the practice, in addition to a royalty fee of two dollars for each denture of six or more teeth. Bacon began suing dentists who refused for patent infringement, and from almost the beginning received favorable court rulings, obtaining judgments and injunctions. In 1866 he sued a slew of America's most respected dentists. The profession responded by forming the American Dental Protective Society and appealing for funds to mount a legal defense and fight back against Bacon:

Brethren of the dental profession throughout the United States . . . The cause that we have undertaken is that of a great profession against a great monopoly. We appeal to you, to leave nothing undone toward the overthrow of these illegal claims, and to secure to the dental profession for all time, the free use of all Vulcanizable compounds.

But the dentists continued to suffer legal setbacks. Thousands of dentists grumbled and paid the licensing fee, although many others turned to the clandestine use of Vulcanite. Company sleuths crossed the country trying to ferret out these rubber robbers. Announcements like the one in the *Jacksonville, Illinois Journal* of the era gave fair warning to one and all:

> Drs. Widenham and Cary are duly authorized licensees in Morgan County for using Vulcanite bases for mounting artificial teeth. We warn all dentists infringing on our patent and all persons employing them that they will be prosecuted to the full extent of the law.

Although the suits were filed in the name of the Goodyear Dental Vulcanite Company, those in the profession knew who the real villain was: "Josiah Bacon, the active and engineering Mephistopheles of this whole skinning raid upon the dentists," in the words of one dental journal.

Samuel S. White, of the S. S. White Dental Company, became a leading voice in the crusade against Bacon. The company's industry organ, *Dental Cosmos,* closely reported on the trials and tribulations. Plans were made to mount an appeal to the Supreme Court challenging the validity of the patent. But in 1872, Bacon's opponents learned a dentist who'd been successfully sued had filed an appeal with the Supreme Court, and that it was dismissed, effectively blocking further appeal against the patent.

A subsequent investigation revealed the appeal was a sham, engineered by Bacon for the purpose of being dismissed. The facts were brought before the justices, and for the first time in its history, the Supreme Court reversed itself, and vacated its affirmation of the lower court's ruling, citing the appeal's collusive nature.

This didn't stop Bacon. It only meant now he had to keep going after dentists one at a time, which he continued to do with relish, using methods detailed in this contemporary newspaper account:

> He employed spies in nearly every city in the Union and paid them liberally to hunt down delinquent dentists. He could well afford to do this for the profits which the Vulcanite Company

derived from the royalty amounted to a princely income. One of his favorite methods of discovering infringements . . . was to employ a beautiful young lady, whom no dentist would suspect. She would call upon the dentist and have him take an impression, to be reproduced in rubber. She was liberal with her money, and only particular on the one subject of the rubber. This once obtained, she had all the evidence requisite to enable Bacon to bring suit . . . servants of dentists were bribed; next door neighbors were questioned, and intimidation was often resorted to.

When an appeal finally did make its way to the Supreme Court again in 1877, the decision went to Bacon—as did all the money he collected in his lawsuits. Now he was more aggressive than ever in his suing and screwing of the dental profession. In 1879 he set off on a cross-country business trip, filing lawsuits all the way from Boston to San Francisco. He arrived in the City by the Bay with a list of about forty dentists he planned to sue. One in particular he was looking forward to seeing—at least in court: Dr. Samuel P. Chalfant. Chalfant had been sued by Bacon at least twice before, each time abandoning his practice rather than pay a licensing fee, and had moved to San Francisco to get as far away from Bacon as possible.

In those days having a case heard didn't take the years it does now; justice was swift even if it didn't always seem like justice. Trials were even held on Saturdays. That's when Chalfant had his day in court to answer charges of patent infringement. Chalfant was found guilty. The following day, Easter Sunday, the despondent dentist went to Bacon's hotel room and drilled him with lead.

BACON'S SHOOTING DEATH brought an end to heavy-handed denture-patent enforcement. When the patent on Vulcanite dentures expired in 1881, the company announced it would not seek an extension. The price fell within range of the common toothless person. The era of artificial teeth for the masses had finally arrived. But the low cost of Vulcanite and the simplicity of its use for dental castings proved threatening to some dentists. They complained their skill and craftsmanship could now be duplicated, if not upstaged, by "mere technicians."

In the case of Vulcanite, invention was the mother necessity. The patent fees drove dentists to experiment with other cheap materials that could be formed into reliable dentures. Celluloid was one alternative. Introduced by John Wesley Hyatt in 1869, it was malleable and unencumbered by patents and licenses. However, it tended to turn an unattractive shade of green after extended use, and was prone to warping.

One noteworthy aspect of the celluloid, aside from cosmetic concerns, was its flammability. This would not typically be a concern for a device worn in the oral cavity, but there is reference in the literature to a British gentleman whose celluloid false teeth caught fire when he dozed off with a cigarette between his lips at his club.

By the late 1800s, dentures were made using hinged devices called articulators, which crudely mimicked the movements of the jaws. The plaster casts of the jaws would be set on the articulator so that the dentures would not only fit together, but perform in a more realistic manner.

Vulcanite, meanwhile, remained in use as the primary denture base material until the eve of World War II, despite its reddish brown color. In the ensuing rubber shortage, acrylic resins marched to the forefront as the base material of choice, and remain so today.

False ID

DENTURES AND DETECTIVE work have sometimes gone hand in hand in bringing criminals to justice. Artificial teeth played a major role in solving one of the most celebrated crimes of the nineteenth century, the murder of George Parkman. The rich, generous, and respected Boston physician failed to return home for dinner in November of 1849. A large search was mounted. Twenty-eight thousand handbills were printed and a $4,000 reward offered for his recovery, dead or alive. The first clue was found by a janitor at the Massachusetts Medical College (now the Harvard Medical School): calcined bones, a dental prosthesis, and melted gold were found in an assay furnace. Mutilated human remains were found in a tea chest. All were in a chemistry department laboratory directed by John White Webster. Webster was arrested and indicted for the willful and premeditated murder of Parkman. Identifying the remains as Dr. Parkman would be crucial. The artificial teeth were the only useable evidence.

The trial quickly established that Dr. Parkman had lent Webster money since 1842 and repeated requests for repayment were ignored. It was alleged Webster lured the doctor to the lab under pretense of paying off part of his debts, where he assaulted and killed Parkman with a jackknife, then mutilated and destroyed all identifiable body parts.

The parade of witnesses was a Who's Who of dentistry. Nathan Cooley Keep (1800–1875), Dr. Parkman's dentist, identified blocks of mineral teeth recovered from the furnace as those he made for Parkman. His identification turned Keep into a household name. W. T. G. Morton, who was himself the subject of the anesthesia controversy, testified for the defense, disputing the provenance of the teeth. Charles Thomas Jackson (1805–1850) MD, Morton's later nemesis, testified as to the amount of gold (173.65 grains) recovered from the assay furnace. Even professor of anatomy Oliver Wendell Holmes appeared as a witness.

After one hundred twenty-one witnesses (sixty-four prosecution, fifty-seven defense) the case went to the jury. It took them three hours to return a guilty verdict. Webster was sentenced to death by hanging and executed in August of 1850. Before execution he repented for his crime, and apologized for having accused the janitor who found the remains of complicity in the disappearance.

Had the teeth not been in the cranium, but exposed, they would have burned up in the furnace, too, and with it all hope of justice for Parkman.

As discussed, Paul Revere used a prosthetic device to make a posthumous identification. A similar feat had reportedly been performed in India in 1194 when the body of a raja defeated in battle was "recognized by his false teeth."

Methods of using the teeth for identification were standardized with the introduction of odontoscopy to forensic dentistry in 1926 in Vienna by Soerup. His method was based on taking direct imprints of the teeth on paper, and would be used to identify otherwise identifiable victims of crimes and catastrophes.

Plaster dental casts have been used at least once not to prove, but to disprove an identity—that of the self-styled Anastasia, who claimed to be the daughter of Nicholas, Czar of Russia. Following their execution in Ekaterinburg, stories circulated that one of the four daughters, Anastasia, had escaped the slaughter. The woman purporting to be Anastasia had a long career in this role, playing both in Europe and New York. However, the Romanov family's Russian dentist, Kostritzky, had preserved plaster casts of each child's jaw, and was able to demonstrate that the real Anastasia had a totally different alignment of the teeth in her lower jaw than did her impostor.

8

X-Ray Martyrs

Toxic, Addictive, Deadly, and Disgusting
Substances Turned on the Teeth

W E HAVE SEEN HOW THE ORAL CAVITY REFLECTED THE INSULTS of a cavalcade of mechanical incompetence and technological shortcomings. We have observed the ancients' misapplication and abuse of a panoply of caustic and corrosive materials turned toothward. Thankfully, arsenic, strong acids, and the like have long ago been removed from the dentist's formulary. Yet progress sometimes bears bitter—or poisonous—fruit, and recent dental history has produced hazards no tooth demon could have dreamed up. In some instances, dentists themselves have been cast in the role of victim of these substances. Others ensnared our youngest and most innocent dental patients.

A Juvenile Preoccupation

IN 1790, JOHN Greenwood, esteemed member of the renowned family of American dentists, placed a notice in the *New York Daily Advertiser* addressed to "Parents & Guardians." The ad stated that from henceforth, Greenwood would, for an annual fee, provide ongoing care to children's teeth, "to give every one an opportunity to be benefited by him. For four Children or upwards, in one family, per year, one guinea. For one child per year, ten shillings, to be paid when the year is out from the time of entering."

It was a defining moment of pediatric dentistry, crystallizing a

174 • James Wynbrandt

growing awareness of the special needs of juvenile patients and the profit potential they represented. By the mid-1800s, concern with youngsters' oral health would result in the institutionalized mutilation of their gums and by the end of the century would create an epidemic of precocious addiction and overdoses. These extreme measures and medicines were deemed warranted by the dangers of the medical crisis they were employed to alleviate: teething.

Today it is simply an uncomfortable rite of passage—for parent as well as child. But in the mid-1800s teething was considered a disease, one that needed to be cured. The eruption of the teeth was seen as a dangerous process that, if untreated, led to a legion of health problems.

Dentist Samuel X. Radbill gravely noted "parents could not rejoice until the child had safely survived the period of dentition." One British expert warned "the period of dentition is one of more than ordinary peril to the child." Another expressed concern for "the distressing symptoms which children suffer while cutting their teeth—viz., Feverish Heats, Fits, Convulsions, Sickness of Stomach and Debility, accompanied by Relaxation of the Bowels, and pale and green motions, or Inflamation of the Gums."

The preferred instrument of treatment was the lance, wielded freely by dentists (and physicians) to cure pediatric health problems.

In an issue of the *American Journal of Dental Science* in 1853, a dentist reported that a young patient of nine to ten months old exhibited strabismus (crossed eyes). The dentist was intent on lancing the gums to relieve the problem but the mother refused. Alas! The child died within a week, according to the writer.

Despite the howling protests of youngsters, dentists and doctors lanced on, convinced of the wisdom of their therapy. A letter in *Dental Cosmos,* from 1870, on "Lancing the Gums in Dentition," seems a study in self-delusion and cruelty:

> There are three objections to scarifying the gums: First, the pain and struggling to the child; second, the increased difficulty of teeth arising from the cicatrix [scar tissue]; third, the danger of hemorrhage.
>
> As for pain, it is trifling, and unworthy of notice. The consequent relief is much more than sufficient to counterbalance the pain. Often the itching of the gums is so intolerable that

the impression of the lancet is agreeable. I have known a child to close its jaws on the instrument and press it into the gum with evident satisfaction.

The struggling of the child, and its fright, are of greater importance, especially if the operation be bunglingly done, as is often the case. There is but one right way of doing it. Take your seat behind the child as it rests on the nurse's lap in a proper light, and placing your knees toward its back, draw its head down between your knees. Let the nurse hold the infant's hands. What with your knees and your two hands, the head is now completely under your control. Grasp it between your two palms, and as it opens its mouth to cry, thrust one of two fingers of the left hand in its mouth to keep the jaws apart, and use the lancet with the other hand. By this method you have the most perfect command of the head and can cut exactly in the spot and to the extent you desire. I am thus precise in the description because I have so often seen the operation so awkwardly undertaken as to fail of its purpose, and to endanger serious wounding of the child's mouth.

There was an easier way to treat what was surely the most troubling symptom of the disease: the crying and wails that the discomfort provoked in teething tots. A variety of tonics and syrups brought quick, quieting relief. They began to appear in the late 1700s in England. The formulas for some of the concoctions were patented. Others claimed to be. Soon all packaged elixirs came to be known as patent medicines. And all were either of dubious value or outright dangerous due to harmful or addictive ingredients.

Dr. Godfrey's General Cordial and Dalby's Carminative were two medicines widely used to treat teething children, often with fatal results, according to contemporary accounts. In 1776 an English observer wrote:

Those convulsions which carry off thousands of infants every year are chiefly owing to the brutality and laziness of nurses who are for ever pouring Godfrey's Cordial down their little throats, which is a strong opiate and in the end as fatal as arsenic.

Even babies who'd built up a tolerance thanks to their habits weren't safe. Dr. Godfrey's General Cordial was found to have a "dangerous opium variance" among various compared samples.

Besides opium, morphine and high concentrations of alcohol were popular active ingredients. The introduction of hypodermic injection of soluble salts of opium alkaloids, first demonstrated in England in 1855, would help illuminate the addictive power of these narcotics. In the United States, society began to awaken to the dangers of opium in the 1860s. By the 1870s opium addiction was a widely recognized problem. Importation of crude opium grew steadily, reaching a per capita peak in the United States in 1896 as patent medicines proliferated. Dr. Drake's Universal Pain Conqueror promised to cure toothaches, "the hell of all disease," in three minutes. Competitors quickly promised relief in one minute. In 1898 heroin was introduced as a cough suppressant.

It was a golden age of drug abuse. The hugely successful Mrs. Winslow's Soothing Syrup, peddled to "quiet fretful children during teething," was a cocktail of morphine and alcohol. Heroin was the active ingredient in Bayer Cough Medicine. Coca Cola took its name from the cocaine that put the twitch in "soda jerks." But as the new century approached, public abhorrence of addiction grew, fueled by what one chronicler called "a wave of moral revulsion."

The "Great Patent Medicine Era" which began in the United States at the end of the Civil War, ended on January 1, 1907, with the passage of the Pure Food and Drug Act, outlawing the misbranding or adulteration of all foods and drugs manufactured in or shipped within the United States. It also helped remove other dangerous dental products, like electric toothbrushes said to be "so electrically primitive, they threatened fatal shock." But as for actually banning addictive drugs or the habit-forming teething medicines, it was just an Act. Narcotics remained a staple of over-the-counter drugs.

During the second decade of the 1900s a crusade against "baby-killing medicines" began. Critics called for an opiate ban. But as one patent-medicine advocate noted, "Medicine would be a one-armed man if it did not possess" the powerful but addictive active ingredients.

Manufacturers began to voluntarily reduce the amount of morphine and opium. Mrs. Winslow's Soothing Syrup had 0.4 grains of morphine per ounce in 1908 and 0.16 grains per ounce in 1911. A ceiling was placed on the amount of opium that could be put in products, finally ending with the Harrison Act of 1914, which banned narcotics altogether.

Mrs. Winslow's Syrup dropped the word "Soothing" from its name and morphine from its ingredients, though the packaging remained the same. Such was the sensitivity to its past that the company sued a motion-picture producer in 1921, claiming a caption in his silent film had held the product "to public scorn and derision." The movie had portrayed an explosion that rendered several people unconscious. The text read, "As a sleep producer, Charlie's incense has it all over Mrs. Winslow's Soothing Syrup."

Raising Cain and Numbing Pain

EVEN AS PRECOCIOUS junkies were nodding out on opiates in the latter 1800s, a new anesthetic, derived from a South American shrub, was stimulating interest in the medical community. A young German chemist, Albert Niemann, had succeeded in isolating the principal alkaloid from the leaves of the South American coca bush in 1860. He suggested calling the alkaloid "Cocain."

In 1864 von Schroff observed the anesthetic effects of cocaine on the tongue. Peruvian general surgeon Thomas Moerno y Maiz suggested its anesthetic properties four years later. One of the early boosters of cocaine's medicinal application was Sigmund Freud, who believed it was a miraculous answer to a variety of behavioral and medical problems. Freud encouraged Dr. Carl Koller, a Vienna physician, to experiment with its analgesic properties.

In 1884 Koller made a historic address at the Ophthalmologic Congress at Heidelberg, where he demonstrated the local anesthetic effects of cocaine by administering a 2 percent solution to the eye of his subject. Following Koller's announcement, experimentation with cocaine proceeded rapidly. The localized effect of the anesthesia was its major attraction. And the ideal delivery vehicle was available, thanks to the refinement of hypodermic injection. In a strange twist of fate, the guinea pig for cocaine's first application in surgery would be a dentist.

In 1884, A few weeks after Koller's demonstration, William Stewart Halsted, MD, of New York, injected cocaine, supplied by Lehn & Fink Co., into the lower jaw of said dentist, then extracted a tooth painlessly. The dentist reported the event in a letter to *Dental Cosmos*:

This evening, Dr. Halsted gave me an injection of seventeen minims . . . in three minutes there was numbness and tingling of the skin . . . in six minutes, there was complete anesthesia of the left half of the lower lip. . . . A pin thrust completely through the lip caused no sensation whatever . . . hard blows upon the teeth with the back of a knife caused no sensation . . ."

This was the first practical use of local anesthetics for dental treatment. It seemed superior to the imprecise effects of laughing gas. Soon cocaine was in wide use as an anesthetic by dentists and physicians. Cocaine toothache drops and other cocaine-based remedies also became popular. As an additional benefit, the drug had euphoric side effects.

Yet the medical community was learning cocaine was far from an ideal anesthetic. As experimentation and application increased, cocaine's dark side was exposed. It was chemically unstable, expensive, toxic, and could cause "sloughing," or necrosis of tissue. In addition to the dangers it presented to patients, many dentists and physicians succumbed to the ravages of addiction. Members of Halsted's staff, even Halsted himself, were not deaf to its siren call. In a letter to noted physician Sir William Osler in 1919, Halsted reported three of his assistants "acquired the cocaine habit in the course of our experiments on ourselves." Ultimately, "They all died without recovery from the habit."

According to the *Journal of the American Dental Association,* "Dr. Halsted did not escape addiction, either, although it is believed that he overcame that addiction before his death in 1922." By that time he'd been named chief of the surgical staff at Johns Hopkins University Hospital. In the final year of his life, the National Dental Association presented a plaque to Dr. Halsted at a banquet given by the Maryland Dental Association. "To Dr. William S. Halsted from the National Dental Association. In grateful recognition of his original research and discoveries upon which the teaching of local and neuroregional anesthesia in oral and dental practice now rests."

Despite the dangers, due to a lack of suitable substitutes, cocaine remained in wide use by dentists until early in the twentieth century. Its replacement appeared in 1905: Novocain. Novocain had the pain-killing power of cocaine without its addictive or destructive side effects.

Not a perfect anesthetic—and not the same as the Novocain patients receive today—it was nonetheless the first in a series of nonaddictive anesthetics that finally delivered painless dentistry without fear of dependency, such as tropacocaine, eucaine A and eucaine B, butyn, alipin, stovaine, apothesine, and monocaine. Without the trials and missteps with cocaine, who can say if these injectible local anesthetics would have been developed?

Cocaine's withdrawal from accepted use has not ended the dental problems associated with its use, as a report from a pair of Boston dentists in the 1980s indicates:

> Recently, we treated several patients who had acute pain of sudden onset in the mucosal tissues surrounding their maxillary and mandibular anterior teeth. Clinical examination disclosed that the gingival tissues surrounding these teeth were grossly inflamed, gingival bleeding was profuse, and the epithelium had desquamated in several areas. The symptoms were confusing and nonspecific, and mimicked a number of acute diseases of the oral mucosa, such as necrotizing gingivitis (Vincent's disease) and herpetic gingivostomatitis of erosive lichen planus. Careful questioning, however, showed that all these patients were cocaine abusers who were in the habit of rubbing cocaine powder on the gingiva. Apparently, "snorting" cocaine in the conventional way had caused such unpleasant side effects (epistaxis, perforated nasal septums) that they had transferred its use to the oral mucosa.

While Johnny-come-lately cocaine was losing its allure in the clinical setting, one of the first and most toxic of medicinal poisons retained a position of prominence in dentistry: mercury.

Mercury Rising

THE USE OF mercury and a belief in its special powers can be seen as far back and away as 4500 B.C. China, where alchemist Ko Hung avowed that if one held mercury in his hands, "evil spirits would be kept away." History records that Hung ended his days suffering from severe chronic mercury toxicity.

An element commonly seen in thermometers in its silver-white liquid form, mercury vaporizes at temperatures as low as 10 degrees Fahrenheit. The vapor is colorless and odorless, is readily absorbed by the blood and evenly distributes in the brain, kidney, heart, lungs, and liver. However, it demonstrates a predilection for collecting in the central nervous system, from which elimination is very slow.

Mercury was used by Greek, Roman, and Arabian physicians. It was a staple ingredient in ointments used to treat parasitic diseases, skin conditions, and disorders of the phallus and testicles. For cosmetic purposes, it found its way into tattoos, in the form of mercury sulfide (cinnabar). Queen Nefertiti of Egypt used it in hers.

No doubt its deleterious side effects were noted by some who came in contact with the substance on a regular basis or in contact with anyone who did. The first description of occupational mercury poisoning found in print is in a 1473 book on goldsmithery, where mercury was used to extract gold from other minerals. But health concerns be damned, half a century later, in 1530, another medical use for mercury was discovered: treatment for syphilis. By the following century some realized the treatment could be worse than the disease, though mercury remained a popular treatment in many places until 1910 when arsenicals (also poisonous) proved their efficacy. Mercury, or mercurous chloride, was also the active ingredient in calomel, used as a topical treatment for skin conditions. In powdered form it was used in small doses for ulcers and skin rashes.

Until its use was banned in their businesses in 1941, the fur and felt industries were major sources of occupational mercury poisoning, which of course was the source of the saying, "mad as a hatter."

Health hazards for dentists and patients have been a topic of concern since the 1830s when mercury-based amalgams were introduced. Soon the literature was documenting suspected cases of so-called "amalgam-related illness," helping fuel the amalgam war that raged across the United States. These concerns were largely quieted with the introduction of better amalgams. In recent years, concerns have arisen anew, with reports linking amalgam fillings to neurological illness and multiple sclerosis.

Mercury poisoning or intoxication results from cumulative exposure. Muscular tremors are the first observable sign, initially seen perhaps in the handwriting. It can progress to a multisymptomatic illness characterized by fatigue, insomnia, depression, headache, slurred speech, and a host of peculiar psychic disturbances called "erthism," bouts of self-consciousness, timidity, embarrassment with insufficient reason, resentment of criticism, anxiety, and irritability or excitability. In more advanced cases, hallucinations and memory loss may be present. Intoxication can produce a complete personality change in the affected individual. But wait, there's more: other symptoms include loss of appetite and nausea, lack of concentration, edema (swelling) of the face and legs, excess salivation, metallic taste and foul breath. Gingivitis, recession of the gums, and mobility of the teeth are also common. Once exhibited, owing to the persistence of mercury in the body tissues, symptoms can last for years.

Currently, over 4 million pounds of mercury per year are used in the United States, with over 210,000 pounds used by dentists—about two-and-one-half pounds each on the average. And what of dentists' own exposure? Recent surveys have found at least 10 percent of dental offices in the United States have ambient mercury levels above the National Institute for Occupational Safety and Health recommendations. Blood and urinalysis of dentists attending professional meetings have found from 50 percent to 70 percent of those tested had above-normal levels of mercury. Inhalation of vapors is the dentists' primary source of mercury poisoning, and secondarily direct absorption from handling mercury-tainted compounds.

"No longer can the dental profession ignore the problem of mercury contamination in the dental office," intoned the *Journal of the American Dental Association* in 1976. Fortunately, today devices like the Mercury Vapor Sniffer, Mercury Vapor Meter, Mercury Vapor Monitor, Mercury Vapor Analyzer, and the Mercury Vapor Detector can sniff out the problem.

Radiating Optimism

THE 1895 DISCOVERY of X rays by Wilhelm Conrad Roentgen in Wurzburg, Germany, was a landmark in modern science. His dramatic announcement that these invisible beams could penetrate solid objects challenged accepted scientific wisdom of the day and spurred a whirlwind of research. Within two weeks, radiation was being misused in dental research, as the powerful rays were aimed at the oral cavity.

The first radiographs, or X-ray photos of the teeth, were made early in 1896 by physicist Walter Konig in Frankfurt. Only days later, it is believed, Otto Walkhoff, a dentist in Braunschweig, duplicated the feat with the help of a local physicist, Friedrich Giesel.

These experiments were performed without regard for the effects of exposure to these harmful emissions. The headlong rush to research produced a pantheon of ray-crazy casualties who would come to be known as "X-ray martyrs," in addition to an untold number of highly irradiated patients. But in those early days, the excitement of discovery amid the heady fin de siècle atmosphere swept aside concern and caution. Nearly every laboratory had a Ruhmkorff Coil and a Crooke's tube, the basic equipment required to construct an X-ray machine, and professors were soon demonstrating the amazing perspicacity of the miraculous rays, captured in astonishing photographs.

By the spring of 1896, X-ray machines were coming on line for both research and clinical use. They were crude devices. Variations in the character and power of the X-ray emissions were controlled by a rheostat, which was manually adjusted. The accepted method was called "setting the tube," holding the fluoroscope in one hand while placing the other over the tube. The rheostat controlling the amount of radiation was adjusted according to how well the bones of the hand appeared on the screen. Just the right amount of X-ray penetration was needed. The hand was only exposed for a few seconds, but the cumulative impact would ultimately manifest itself in painful and malignant cancerous lesions on this fraternity of doomed dentists and physicians.

The X-Ray Martyrs

THE FIRST AMERICAN book on X rays appeared in 1896, written by William James Morton, the son of pioneer anesthetist and disgraced dentist William T. G. Morton. He told a dental meeting in April of that year that "the X ray more than rivals your exploring mirror, your probe, your most delicate sense of touch, and your keenest powers of hypothetical diagnosis."

A photograph of the author shows him working with an engineer preparing to take an X ray, fluoroscoping their own hands, unaware of the fatal consequences this experimentation would have for many of its pioneers.

By July, William H. Rollins had invented an intraoral fluroscope.

That same month Dr. Charles Edmund Kells Jr. (1856–1928) gave the first clinic in the United States on the use of X rays in dentistry. Kells had taken the first radiographs of teeth in the United States that spring. A leading dental pioneer of the day, Kells would become the most noted of the X-ray martyrs.

Born in New Orleans, the son of a successful dentist, from an early age he witnessed dangers of dentistry, as his account of an extraction observed in his youth illustrates.

> The patient was seated in the chair, and besides the ordinary gas jet in the room, a candle was held by someone in order to light up the mouth. The ether spray was started [for anesthesia], and the first thing the dentist knew, he saw everything enveloped in flame. He was "scared to death," as the saying is, and the candle holder "liked to have dropped dead with fright," and started to back away from the chair.
>
> As soon as the candle was removed a little distance, the blaze went out—it was the vapor of the ether that had caught fire.
>
> Then composure was regained, and the operation was concluded (more carefully, as far as the candle was concerned) satisfactorily.
>
> Meanwhile, the patient had never "batted an eye." When all was over, the dentist began complimenting the patient upon his nerve upon not being frightened by the fire. "Fire? What fire?" "Why, when the flame shot up." "Oh, I thought that was part of the process."

Kells was familiar with frightful dental practices of a more prosaic nature, as well, such as those of a California dentist who employed a particularly painful method of cleansing putrescent root canals. "His method of removing pulp from a singe-rooted tooth was by 'knocking it out' with an orangewood stick and phenol. This sounds atrocious, but, as a matter of fact, was not always so. However, I reckon only those of us who did it successfully will believe that statement. Remember, please, there was no such thing as 'local anesthesia' in those days."

Some of Kells own practices were atrocious, though not in the dental department. He was a committed racist, or an "unreconstructed Johnny Reb" as he wrote in his autobiography, *Three Score and Ten*.

He joined the infamous White League at age seventeen. Years later he was still kicking himself for being absent the day his comrades went on a bloody rampage against reconstructionist officials that "wiped out the carpetbag despots," as he put it. Though he was happy about the results—"and the white people resumed the reins of government"— his absence remained a personal disappointment throughout his life— "and I missed it all. Just my luck."

Electrifying Developments

KELLS WENT TO New York Dental College in 1876 and became friendly with technicians from Thomas Edison's Menlo Park laboratory. He would often hang around the lab, observing the work and experiments in progress. He saw some of the first electric incandescent lamps, sparking his own lifelong interest in electricity, electromagnetism, and its application in dentistry. The horizons must have seemed limitless. Electricity had the power to transform dentistry. When the Edison Electric Light Company began to supply power to major users in New Orleans, Kells signed up for service. He wired his office himself and connected it to the power grid outside his office, becoming the city's first dentist using street current to power his electrical dental apparati.

The electricity seemed to unleash an inventive energy in the doctor. Among his inventions was an automatic electric suction pump which drained saliva, thereby keeping the mouth dry during dental procedures. It was widely adapted by dentists, and soon found its way into surgical operating rooms as well, replacing the use of surgical sponges for mopping up bodily fluids. Ultimately Kells acquired thirty patents for devices including an electric thermostat, fire extinguisher and alarm, automobile starter, drinking fountain, and an electromagnetic clock.

Yet even as Kells rushed headlong into this brave new world of electricity, others questioned the safety of the forces dentistry was harnessing, the effects of exposure to electricity and the dangers of electrocution. The doctor was cognizant of these anxieties, and apparently entertained doubts himself. "The chair" was already frightening to many patients. The prospect that it, too, would have current running through it must have raised fears even before electrified seats became a favored method of execution. Kells's own concerns can be read in a letter to M. J. Grier, a prominent physician and editor of the *Dental Cosmos*. The communiqué was sent concurrently with Kells's inquiry to the S.S. White Dental Manufacturing Company, asking about their ability to make electric dental equipment for him.

"Dear Doctor," Kells wrote, "Knowing your long experience and thorough familiarity with the uses of electricity in medicine and in the arts, I venture to ask a frank opinion from you as to the risks of whatever kind you recognize in the application of the arc and the incandescent currents to the various motors in use by dentists and in such other uses as the said currents are employed for in dental and medical offices."

Dr. Grier responded cautiously:

> The use of commercial lighting current, as shown by the apparatus exhibited by you, to give the light and heat needed and to actuate the motors employed in the dental office, opens up a fascinating and almost unlimited field of application. . . . Unfortunately, these currents, especially the light arc, possess an electromotive force and strength far beyond the needs of the case, and therein lies the risk of their employment. . . . THE POSSIBLE TRANSFERENCE OF THE CURRENT FROM THE APPARATUS TO THE PERSON OF THE OPERATOR OR THE PATIENT. . . . Accidents will happen with the best-regulated systems. Admitting that within the office every precaution is taken to insure the greatest exemption from danger, there are many external causes beyond the control of the most careful and skillful persons, such as tornadoes, storms in winter abrading the insulation and breaking the wires, grounding perhaps a high potential circuit and carrying it directly into the office. The same may happen during thunderstorms; and, in cases of fire, heat and falling walls may produce similar results. Other causes might be mentioned, but perhaps enough has been said to direct the attention of the profession generally to the possible dangers attending the introduction and use for motors of electric currents as furnished by the light and power companies.
>
> Very truly yours,
> M. J. Grier, MD

Kells noted another threat to practitioners emanating from dental offices—not their own, but the offices of an expanding population of dental specialists. It was the specialists themselves. Their very existence endangered the poor "family dentist." "The 'Soul of the Dentist,'" Kells proclaimed, "is being dimmed." Too many procedures were being turned over to niche practitioners. "And your erstwhile family dentist," he asked rhetorically, "where does he come in?" A lament cum poem he wrote on the subject provided the answer:

> *Tooth is to be extracted? Exodontist.*
> *Teeth regulated? Orthodontist.*
> *Pyorrhea? Periodontist.*
> *Teeth need cleaning? Dental Hygienist.*
> *Root canals to be filled? Pathodontist.*
> *Baby's tooth hurts? Pedodontist.*
> *Plate to be made? Prosthodontist.*
> *Nothing the matter? Impossible! Radiodontist.*
> *Tooth to be filled? Oh what luck! Home at last!*

X Marks the Spot

DESPITE HIS DOUBTS about specialists and electricity, Kells appeared oblivious to the very real danger that would eventually claim his life.

In 1896, Tulane University gave a demonstration of X rays, and Kells was of course in attendance. A hand was photographed with an X-ray device, with an exposure of twenty minutes. The results astonished Kells. Knowing the professor, Kells asked for a machine, expressing a desire to take "pictures of the teeth." By April or May of 1896 he had his device and was taking dental X rays.

In July the Southern Dental Association gathered in Ashville, North Carolina, and Dr. Kells gave a demonstration of the Roentgen ray phenomenon. He set up his apparatus and allowed attendees to come forth and view the effects of its penetrating rays. The display created a sensation.

"There was a charity ball going on that night which came near proving to be a failure as the patrons deserted the ball room, crowded in to take their turns before the machine and view the bones of their hands, contents of their purses, and so on," he recalled. "The members of our own association had to struggle along in the line awaiting their turns."

"No one took any skiagrams from living subjects prior to this date," he said. However, the crowds were so large it proved impossible to make skiagrams of the teeth.

Kells began integrating X rays into his dental practice. It had taken twenty minutes of exposure for a hand, but with an improved tube the area around a molar could be done in fifteen minutes. In 1903 Kells established the New Orleans X-Ray Laboratory, located in the same building as his offices. The announcement of the opening carried several illustrations of X-ray photographs: the head of a living subject with a bullet in it, a foot with a needle in it, a hip bone and a lower molar with a diagnostic wire in it. This was, he said, "Undoubtedly the first illustration of its kind ever published."

Other pioneering dental X-ray experiments were performed by practitioners including Weston A. Price in 1901, Sinclair Tousey in 1905, and M. L. Rhein in 1911.

In 1913 Kells installed the first commercial X-ray unit made especially for use in dentistry. But after some dozen years of exposure, Dr. Kells had developed malignant growths on his left hand. It was the beginning of years of agony. He later noted the dangers of radiation had been recognized even before then, and no prudent operator would hold a film in the mouth of his patient or in any way expose his hands to the direct rays. Rollins had noted burns on the skin of his hands following his early experiments, and in 1901 suggested operators should wear the "most nonradiable material" possible when using the equipment, and that patients should likewise be covered with radiation-proof material.

Early X-ray machines could be dangerous for more than their radiation. As Dr. Grier had indicated in his response to Kells in *Dental Cosmos,* the electricity that powered these contraptions could also be hazardous. The exposed high-tension wires of these devices caused several serious accidents and a few fatalities by themselves. In one such incident, a runaway horse outside the office window caught the attention of a woman about to have an X ray taken. She pointed excitedly at the runaway steed as the dentist was about to engage the electricity. He turned involuntarily to see what she was pointing at and came in contact with the exposed electrical wires as he pressed the button. The jolt of electricity threw him into the wall across the room, fracturing his skull. Such exposed wires were not eliminated until the appearance of the first "safety" X-ray machine, produced in 1923.

Dr. Kells suffered through the slower, more insidious effects of the equipment's misuse. He underwent some ten to twelve operations on his hand in the ensuing years. (He lost count of the exact number, he said.) He described all of them as minor, though each time he lost portions of his fingers. He used the leeches he recommended for stubborn tooth infections on his unhealing wounds, but they proved ineffectual. Exposure to radium, another toxic radioactive element was apparently part of the therapy.

When one more cancerous ulcer appeared on a finger, Dr. Kells began to despair of ever finding a cure. Then he heard about a therapy recommended by a "very well-known advocate of the ultraviolet ray as produced by a quartz tube." At the urging of this advocate, Dr. Kells underwent ultraviolet ray treatment, exposing his affected hand to strong doses of ultraviolet radiation—more X rays—three times a week. Soon the ulcer grew worse. He underwent a series of more operations, each time losing more of his hand, then his arm. In unrelenting agony, Kells finally took his own life with a gun. He left a rich legacy of innovation and invention to the dental profession, and a poignant warning about the force that captivated his life and wrought his death:

Friends, I beseech you, beware of the ultraviolet ray.

Focal Infection Hysteria

DESPITE THE PENALTY paid by its pioneers, the X ray proved a powerful dental tool, exposing the oral cavity as it had never been seen before. Anatomical structures and pathological conditions of the teeth and jaw bones stood starkly revealed. From earliest use, one condition it frequently found were pockets of infection beneath the gum.

Soon, "focal infection," as these infected areas were called, became suspects in the causation of a variety of maladies, and not only dental disorders. Afflictions of all organs and extremities were soon being blamed on focal infections, and the X ray was the primary tool for discovering them. The country was swept by what became known as "focal infection hysteria," and once more the rays' use would prove to have damaging consequences.

The roots of the hysteria went back to at least the beginning of the nineteenth century. In 1801, Benjamin Rush, one of the signers of Declaration of Independence and a leading United States physician, published clinical reports on focal infection and its connection to general health. He found removing decayed teeth and clearing up attendant infections could lead to the spontaneous cure of a variety of ailments of unknown origin manifest in other parts of the body. It was not an original idea (Fauchard, for example, had written of the woman whose inexplicable headaches were cured by the removal of carious teeth), but Rush's stature helped give the theory credence.

Regarding his contribution, Rush later wrote, "I have been made happy by discovering that I have only added to the observations of other physicians in pointing out a connection between extraction of decayed and diseased teeth and the cure of general diseases."

Restorative techniques developed in the latter 1800s added to the rate of these infections. Improvements in materials and tools, such as a workable dental cement (introduced in 1869) and an effective foot-operated dental "engine" to power a drill, as Morrison unveiled in 1871, enabled decayed teeth to be restored with crowns. Yet while the work was cosmetically impressive, the hand instruments of the day made proper preparation of the roots virtually impossible. They were typically saved but rarely cleaned and filled. Bremmer explained the results in the *Story of Dentistry*:

> Frequently the teeth under the well-constructed bridges would abscess and develop pus-discharging fistulae, but few dentists were disturbed by these manifestations. When a patient expressed some apprehension about tenderness over the root ends, or the flow of some exudate from the gums, he was usually told not to worry about it. The fact that teeth were intimately connected with the bloodstream and the nervous system seemed to have escaped the attention not only of the dentist but of the physician as well.

The British, who had been upstaged by their upstart American cousins in dentistry, launched an attack against such practices in 1911.

Physician William Hunter publicly accused "American dentistry" of contributing to the ill health of the populace. He cited case histories of patients bedridden with unexplainable illnesses, some of whom had had extensive restorative dental work, or American dentistry, performed on them. A few of these unfortunates, at his suggestion, reluctantly had the bridges and roots removed. The results? Several began to improve rapidly. The obvious implication? The infection in the tooth roots and the roots of their unexplained illnesses were one in the same. In his attack, Hunter called the bridges "mausoleums of gold over a mass of sepsis."

Soon, medical practitioners from all fields began to consider the teeth's—specifically the pockets of infection around them—effect on health. As much as the roots had been ignored, now they were obsessively considered. Any illness whose cause could not otherwise be identified was now deemed to result from these sites of "focal infection." Alarm reached near-panic proportions. The accepted remedy, for the sake of overall health, was to remove any and all such affected teeth.

X rays could be used to reveal this hidden threat, by seeing beneath the gums, where the infection lurked. However, X-ray photographs of the era were prone to misinterpretation regarding the presence of such pockets. Dentists tended to err on the side of caution. By the 1920s, "focal infection hysteria" stimulated an orgy of extractions. Young, old, robust, weak: Soon all were having their teeth yanked at the first sign of illness. The hysteria resulted in a generation of edentulous adults. Unfortunately these wholesale extractions were usually ineffective in bringing the relief for which they were performed.

A Brush with Disaster

THE PUBLIC IN these less-enlightened times was not even safe from simple dentifrices. Many of the products offered to keep teeth clean contained harsh chemicals or abrasives capable of scouring or eating away tooth enamel with ease.

The first compounds meant for cleaning teeth were not pastes, but powders, and were quite effective. Often made of crushed coral or pumice, their coarse grit scoured away the enamel along with the impurities that discolored the teeth. Remember the results of British dentist Thomas Berdmore's experiments with one typical compound of the day, and the ease with which he stripped off the tooth's hearty white overcoat.

The powders typically made claims to arresting decay, removing tartar and "scurf" and restoring the gums to health, and of course were breathlessly promoted in the most overreaching and unsubstantiated manner. An ad for one, Sozodont, proclaimed, "The daily demand for SOZODONT is a marvel in the annals of toilet requisites. It exceeds that of all other dentifrices combined. This famous article is one of acknowledged merit, and those who once use it will always use it; hence its immense sale.—It is supplied by all Chemists and Perfumers, or direct from the Wholesale agent."

This same product was branded "a most infernal humbug," during an 1866 meeting of the American Dental Association's Committee on Dentifrices, as "it cut teeth like so much acid."

Half a century later the problem was no better. Early in the twentieth century, Pepsodent advertised that the pepsin that gave the product its name removed dental film, "thereby preventing acidity of the mouth, decay and pyorrhea." Not so, said William J. Giles, a professor of chemistry at Columbia University, who analyzed the toothpaste. What he did find was an abrasive "hard and sharp enough to cut glass," along with a conclusion "that Pepsodent is put on the market in utter ignorance of the dental and biochemical principles involved, or with intent to mislead the multitude that may usually be deceived by a plausible advertisement."

In 1909 Giles began studying the composition of tooth powders, pastes, and mouthwashes, condemning the "highfalutin' dupery" he found. In the 1920s he turned his ire on the American Dental Association, criticizing the organization for indifference to fatuous and dangerous nostrums. Still the ADA kept its teeth together and dangerous dentifrices continued to appear. In the mid-1930s, one whitening agent, a product called Tartaroff, contained 1.2 percent hydrochloric acid. It was said to be capable of destroying 3 percent of the tooth's enamel in a single application.

It's a Gag

SOME DEVICES TURNED on the teeth were harmful only to financial health. A variety of quack devices have been used to relieve patients of their money, if not their misery. The rogues' gallery roll call of such gadgets from the world of dentistry includes the Improved Magneto Electric Machine (ca. 1862), the Pratt Battery; the Oxydonor; The Radiolux; Dr. Scott's electric toothbrush (on the market before electricity was invented); Burchell Anodyne Necklace (1807); the violet Ray Machine, and Baunscheidt's Lebenswecker.

Other remedies were merely disgusting and degrading, not deleterious. Folklorists have collected many recommended animal-based cures for toothaches, whose ingredients include ants, beetles, cockroaches, crabs, crayfish and snails, frogs and toads, lizards, newts, salamanders, fish, snakes, birds, rabbits and hares, rodents, hedgehogs, mice, moles, hoofed animals, deer, donkeys and asses, and carnivorous animals. Human excrement and other waste products have also been recommended as ameliorative emollients and toothache remedies.

Today the dental office is much less the minefield than it was in its infancy. But hazards still face the unwary, often from the most innocuous objects. The danger is that they can be—and have been—swallowed. Rubber dam clamps, crowns, gauze pads, rubber plantes, and pieces of plaster are among the objects that have disappeared down patients' throats during treatment. This possibility is probably not considered by most, but it needs to be taken seriously, even if it is just a gag.

Breathing Easy?

MEANWHILE, OLD THREATS crop up anew. Nitrous oxide, for example. Laughing gas was avoided by some practitioners in its early days due to the unpredictability of its effect on patients. These drawbacks were gradually addressed as delivery systems became more sophisticated. But now it is the dentists themselves who may be most at risk, as a result of recreational use of nitrous oxide.

According to concerned professionals, many dentists are known to have "passing paralysis of their legs caused by nitrous oxide abuse." Indeed, the gas has been labeled an "opioid addictive agent," though many dentists are unaware of its potential habit-forming properties due to lack of controls on its use. In one year of the 1980s alone, at least two dentists and one dental student died from nitrous oxide inhalation. Death usually results from blockage of their airways after abusers fall asleep in a dental chair under its influence.

Nonabusive dentists may also be at risk. The affects of habitual exposure to trace levels of the anesthetic gas are poorly understood and documented. An estimated 35 percent of dentists use inhalation sedation techniques. What studies have been done indicate that this population exhibits a higher rate of spontaneous abortions, both among pregnant dentists and among wives of such dentists who were not themselves directly exposed.

And the oldest threat of all remains: quackery. Health experts report that quackery has been on the increase in recent years. Dental education may be partly responsible. Little about the scientific method is taught in dental school. Continuing education, even that offered by respected institutions, may exacerbate the problem by offering pseudoscientific teachings. In the mid-1980s, for example, a five-day course offered through a dental school was described as "an introduction to the philosophy, principles, and practice of osteopathy as it is applied in the cranial field." Another United States university offered CE credits for attending a course that reviewed the "vagrant intraoral galvanic currents" that "disturb the functioning of the central nervous system," thereby unleashing "emotional, intellectual, neurological, digestive, respiratory, cardiovascular, and dermatological" health disturbances.

Among examples of contemporary quackery: a tooth/muscle chart that purports to show the relationship between individual teeth and specific muscles throughout the body. Another trend in quackery identified by dental-care guardians is the linking of disorders of the temporomandibular joint (TMJ), the joint that hinges the jaw to the skull, to overall systemic illnesses.

According to a 1987 article in the *Journal of the American Dental Association*, "Experts also point to the very nature of dental practice as a spawning ground for quackery."

With about seven out of ten dentists working in solo, independent practices, the isolation may lead some practitioners to develop erroneous ideas about a variety of treatments and their efficacy.

9

Disposable Income and Permanent Teeth

A Century of Progress Builds a Dental Bridge to a New Era of Oral Care

A VISIT TO THE DENTIST'S OFFICE TODAY OR A GLANCE INSIDE A medicine cabinet reveals how far oral care has come. In the office, sleek modernism prevails, the functionality reflecting the vision of a pre-cyber society whose eyes have been turned spaceward. Behind our bathroom mirrors crowd the appurtenances of a dentally pampered culture, all manner of brushes, flosses, and home-care tools. Preoccupation with decay and cavities has replaced patients' concerns with life-threatening treatment protocols of yesteryear. Yet who stops to consider this upon hearing the whine of the turbine drill, or when being shown to a contoured dental chair, or viewing cavity-free X-ray slides? A true appreciation for these advances can be difficult to apprehend without familiarity with the evolutionary forces that drove their development.

Watered-Down Decay

IT'S EVERYWHERE—IN the ground, in the air, in your toothpaste, in your face. It's fluoride, and because it's also in the water most Americans now drink, caries and cavities are no longer the scourge they once were. Yet the practice of fluoridating water supplies continues to meet virulent opposition in some quarters, as it has since its introduction.

Fluorine is a common and violently reactive element—so reactive

194

that it's never found alone in its natural state. Rather, it combines with other elements to form fluorides, or salts of fluorine. These compounds are ubiquitous in the soil, air, and the sea. Water flowing over fluoride-bearing minerals absorbs the salts, and hence almost all water from the earth contains fluorides. The amount in a given sample of water depends on the amount of fluorides in the ground it flows over or through.

The first association made between fluoride and teeth is difficult to fix, but by 1874, a German publication for "rational physicians" stated, "As, for a long time, Iron was given for the blood, Calcium and phosphorus for the bones, so has it been successful to add Fluoride to the tooth enamel in a soluble and absorbable form. It is Fluoride that gives hardness and durability to the tooth enamel and protects against caries."

Fluoride pills were reportedly being dispensed in England for this purpose at the time. Dr. Frederick McKay had probably paid little attention to the subject when he arrived in Colorado Springs in 1901, freshly graduated from dental school. He soon noted, however, that many of his patients exhibited a peculiar mottling of their teeth, "minute white flecks, or yellow or brown spots or areas, scattered irregularly or streaked over the surface of a tooth, or it may be a condition where the entire tooth surface is of a dead paper-white, like the color of a china dish."

McKay later moved to St. Louis, and only after he returned to Colorado in 1908 did he pursue the mottled teeth riddle. In 1916 McKay lured esteemed dentist G. V. Black to see the problem—which had been unreported in dental literature—firsthand. Reports of similar occurrences came in from other western towns.

Variations in the level of mottling ultimately led McKay to conclude the quality of the drinking water was a factor, though the causative agent remained unknown. The dental disease was particularly bad in the communities of Oakley, Idaho, and Bauxite, Arizona. McKay recommended changing the communities' water supplies to correct the defect. In 1925 and 1928, respectively, the two towns put his advice into practice, and following the change, no new cases of mottling appeared.

Experts offered theories on what was in the water that caused the problem. Manganese, excessive acidity, and excessive alkalinity of the water were among the offered answers. None of them turned out to be the culprit. A chemist at the Toronto, Ontario Filtration Plant, Frank Hannan, offered yet another hypothesis.

Of the mineral elements at present known to be common to both water and enamel, the chief ones are calcium, phosphorus, and fluorine. For our intake of phosphorus, we are independent of the small proportion found in the water, the same can be asserted of calcium with perhaps a shade less certainty, a dietary deficient in this element being not altogether unusual. But when we consider fluorine, all is at present shrouded in obscurity. The detection and estimation of small traces of fluorine are tedious and troublesome and quite outside the province of the ordinary water-works chemist who has to handle many thousands of samples in a year. . . . Should the incriminated water prove to be all alike fluorine-free, the case for fluorine deficiency will become strong.

McKay carefully considered the conjecture and issued a response. "None of the elements mentioned by Mr. Hannan seem to have any direct possibility of producing a decalcification," McKay wrote.

Hannan had, or course, hit on the correct causative element, but he mistakenly thought the disorder was caused by a fluorine deficiency. It was actually the result of an excess. Meanwhile, town fathers in Bauxite, Arizona, were anxious to absolve aluminum of any culpability. Bauxite is the raw material from which aluminum is made, and Bauxite was a company town, founded by the Aluminum Company of America for its miners. If aluminum was blamed, it would be disastrous for a company whose metal was used in pots and pans. Already some people were criticizing the use of aluminum for cooking, claiming it caused poisoning.

At the company's Pittsburgh laboratories, chemist Dr. H. V. Churchill took up the mystery. His experiments established the link between high fluoride levels and what would come to be called fluorosis, or mottled dental enamel. Independent confirmation came from other studies,

Fluorosis, it was found, caused enamel to weaken. However, it only occurred during calcification of the teeth, a process that lasted until about age twelve. Damage was permanent, though affected teeth were relatively cavity-free. In fact, one study found the lowest incidence of cavities was concentrated in "an endemic fluorisis area," and suggested the fluoride in the water might be the reason.

Ninety-seven percent of tooth enamel is composed of fluoride and hydroxyapatite. These two substances, which have a great affinity for one another, combine to form fluorapatite, a mineral with greater resistance to the ravages of corrosive bacterial by-products than either of its constituent compounds. Ingesting the right amount of fluoride, it was reasoned, might strengthen the teeth from cavities without mottling or weakening the enamel. Now scientists focused on determining the exact effects of varying levels of fluorides.

Over a decade beginning in the late 1930s, thousands of children were examined and water supplies analyzed. Fluroisis was found endemic in 345 locations in twenty-five states. Reports from South America, Australia, Europe, Africa, and Asia revealed the global dimensions of the fluorosis problem. By 1942, a United States Public Health Service dentist, H. Trendley Dean, had demonstrated that one part per million of fluoride in drinking water reduced caries without mottling the teeth. A carefully conducted, yet bold test program was suggested: Public water supplies of selected communities would be fluoridated, and the teeth of a sample of the population's youngsters periodically examined.

Grand Rapids, Michigan, was selected as the site for the first fluoridation program, commencing on January 25, 1945. Aurora, Illinois, and Muskegon, Michigan, were added to the program the same year. Subsequent studies found progressive reduction in the number of decayed, filled, and missing teeth. No other effects other than those on the teeth were reported. The program was expanded and by 1950 over fifty cities were fluoridating their water.

Yet opposition to fluoridation—which had been present from its debut—was growing. Both individuals and groups had protested Grand Rapid's fluoride foray, and the cries of critics swelled during the 1950s. Health-food boosters were among the first to protest, claiming the fluoride would poison the water. Chiropractors protested it as an infringement of personal freedom at the hands of organized medicine; they claimed fluoridation was incompatible with chiropractic nutritional philosophy. Christian Scientists attacked it as forced medication. The John Birch Society linked fluoridation to communism, a conspiratorial plot to poison the water supply. The vocal opposition succeeded in slowing widespread adoption of fluoridation during the 1950s. But by the 1960s, a decade marked by mass ingestion of a multitude of psychoactive chemicals, the battle was only a rearguard action. By the end of the decade the water in almost 3,000 water systems serving 83 million people was being fluoridated.

Some 155 million Americans, about 62 percent of the population, were tapped into fluoridated water supplies at the end of the twentieth century. And today, of course, fluoride is also found in toothpaste and dental treatments. Yet acceptance is still not universal, the fight over fluoride unfinished.

In England, as the twenty-first century dawns, only about 10 percent of the country has fluoridated water supplies—some 5.5 million people. Efforts to increase the percentage have been stymied by fluorophobia. The antifluoride initiative mounted by opponents in one community—Scarborough, in Yorkshire—included giant allegorical sand drawings on a beach of a "Truth Fairy" being harassed by a fluoride-flaunting ogre. In Parliament, a supporter of the opponents labeled fluoride "one of the most toxic poisons known to man," declaring that "a fraction of a teaspoon will kill you."

Joining the battle, the British Fluoridation Society noted opposition was usually greatest in the very places it was acutely needed.

"Our most deprived sections of the community who are most at risk, are more in need of fluoride in the water," a society spokesperson said. "They're not brushing their teeth—or not as frequently as the rest of us."

Even without fluoride, it appears British dental health, long regarded as suspect (if not oxymoronic), has improved. In the early 1980s, a full 28 percent of the adults surveyed by the British Dental Association were missing all their teeth. A decade later, the figure had dropped to 17 percent of adults.

The fight over fluoridation in Great Britain continues. Opponents were buoyed by the case of an eleven-year-old boy who collected $1,600 from Colgate Palmolive, after alleging regular use of the company's Minty Gel toothpaste (containing fluoride) had mottled his teeth and stained them brown. It subsequently turned out that rather than just brushing his teeth with the dentifrice, the youngster had been eating it for years, though his parents had tried unsuccessfully to get him to spit rather than swallow.

The Hole Truth

AS AMERICA BEGAN to season its water with fluoride, dentists were closing in on the secret of the destructive process that fluoridation was intended to obviate.

Dental caries, the decay that resulted in tooth cavities, had afflicted large segments of various populations since Egypt's heyday. And although the evil spirits, worms, and "bad humors" that the ancients had blamed for their dental problems were no longer adequate explanations, no real alternative was offered in their stead. The genesis, or degenesis, of caries, remained a mystery into the twentieth century. Even the causal link between sugar and caries went unrecognized by many while experts debated the source of tooth decay.

During the 1700s and 1800s, one school of thought held that decay began in the pulp and worked its way outward. Another school posited that decay began outside, often at the instigation of acids in foods, and worked its way inward. In 1819 American dentist Levi S. Parmly threw his weight behind this latter theory, writing, "Caries begin on the surface of the teeth by a chemical agency, on those relics of food which accidentally lodged between them . . . causing an active poison which corrodes their structure."

Some suggested sweet, sticky foods played a role, others that a life of luxury and comfort begat caries. Scurvy and medicinal application of mercury were also blamed. Lateral pressure, the force of one tooth pushing against another, was another suspected culprit. Supporters of this theory pointed out that teeth with large spaces between them seldom decayed, ignoring the fact that such wide-open spaces made it more difficult for plaque to build up.

Tartar was believed responsible in some way for the sad progression of declining oral health: gum disease, bone deterioration, loosening, and loss of teeth. The paper "Dental Calculus in the History of Dentistry," originally published in Italian, finds a connection was made between calculus, or tartar, and gingival tissues and gum disease as early as Roman times. Thomas Berdmore suggested cutting out the diseased gum where calculus had damaged it. A painful procedure, he recommended a mouthwash of camphorated opium as a palliative during recuperation.

In 1840, dentist Sir John Tomes observed blue litmus turned red in a cavity, thereby establishing the acidic nature of the corrosive agent.

With improvements in microscopes in the first half of the 1800s, lenses were soon trained on the structures of the oral cavity. In 1867, after discovery of bacteria, Leber and Rottenstein first suggested their possible association with decay. The following year, a suspect wanted for the willful destruction of enamel was identified: *Leptothrix buccalis*. The charges, however, failed to stick. Though exonerated as an innocent bystander, the possible connection of an organism that fit the general description of *L. buccalis* and tooth decay marked a turning point in the investigation.

A breakthrough in the case came with the 1890 publication of Willoughby D. Miller's landmark work, *Micro-organisms of the Human Mouth*. An American dentist and respected professor at the University of Berlin, Miller is credited with discovering the chemicobacterial cause of caries. Miller's research found caries resulted from the initial action of acids arising from the fermentation of food, followed by the action of bacteria attacking the softened tissues. This chemicoparasitic theory, as it is now known, remains the accepted model of the cause and course of caries. But even though the MO was right, there were still no suspects.

The fight against cavities that preoccupied postwar America can be viewed as an extension of the Cold War. The gleaming smile, like our country's bright future, could be undermined and even blighted by an enemy lurking within, working its quiet betrayal unseen. The task of identifying the agents responsible became critical, just as it had been in the witch hunts of the era.

In 1954 a team of scientists led by Frank J. Orland, working in a germ-free laboratory at the University of Notre Dame, proved that dental caries could not form without the presence of microorganisums. But which bacteria are responsible? Only now are investigators naming names. Most suspects live on the wrong side of the plaque, thriving in the sticky yellow film that gives a noirish, smoggy tint to the bad part of the mouth. Here, *Streptococcus mutans* feeds on dissolved sugar, producing acid that demineralizes enamel and dentine. Other monocellular mischief-makers consume organic remains, while the whole community produces toxins that inflame gums and destroy teeth-supporting fiber and bone.

The cause of gum disease likewise remained undiscovered until this era. The misconception that calculus, or tartar, was the cause persisted until the mid-1960s, when bacterial plaque was officially recognized as the cause of gingivitis and periodontitis. But much is still a mystery. Most of the multitude of bacteria believed responsible for gum disease are unidentified. Nor can we answer why the gums of some individuals fall victim to these parasites whereas others do not. Indeed, our knowledge of the decay process remains very much a cavity itself, a dark abyss, ravaged by corrosive ignorance, in great need of filling with facts.

Thus we see in our understanding, as in decay itself, what appears at the outset stable and static is in a state of change, perhaps imperceptible to the unaided eye, but evidencing dramatic shifts over time. This same principle applies to much we can observe in the dental office today, beginning with the physical positioning of dentists themselves.

A Position of Importance

To STAND OR not to stand? After millennia of performing on their feet, the question dentists began to ask themselves during the 1800s seemed every bit as wrenching as Hamlet's conundrum. In surveying the answer the profession forged, one must take into account social forces as well as technological innovations of the era.

Throughout history, while patients' positions had shifted, from the floor to chairs and couches or on their feet, dentists usually stood. Or crouched. But they rarely sat. There were the occasional exceptions of course; the mountebanks who had yanked teeth while astride a horse, or the practitioner who favored sitting on the patient's chest to draw a tooth. Yet as the 1800s advanced, dentists began to take a seat to perform their work. Can it be coincidence that this shift occurred as dentists sought greater respect for their profession, and the industrial revolution created a new working class, one that was poor and stood on its feet all day? For a trade seeking to elevate its status, the similarity between their profession's body language and that of a factory worker would have been unacceptable. This was not simply a matter of standing, we can surmise, but of social standing. Surely some dentists realized in order to raise their profession they would have to lower themselves.

If such a social imperative was at work, one would expect the backlash against standing to be exhibited initially among upper-class practitioners in a country with a rigid social system and a rapidly emerging industrial economy. Thus, one cannot be surprised to learn that Sir John Tomes, British dental pioneer of the mid-nineteenth century (and author of the tome on care of artificial teeth previously cited) was the first to have a dental stool in his operatory, and perhaps the first to sit down while working. His stool, along with dental chair, spittoon, and cabinet, are on display in the museum of the British Dental Association.

Given the emphatic schism with factory work this seating device was no doubt meant to signify, the ample cushion, which has been described even by objective historians as "overstuffed," is noteworthy. This was a gentleman's profession, the stool seems to say, as far from tedious industrial toil as could be imagined.

By the 1870s commercially made dental stools were available and refinements were being added, as with the Dr. I. W. Lyon Improved Adjustable Stool of 1876, used by many "leading" dentists, according to the S. S. White catalog. Yet ambivalence about the new position remained. The popular Morrison dental chair, patented in 1887, was said to owe its success in part to "its extraordinary range of vertical movement . . . the dentist can operate with equal convenience whether sitting or standing."

Despite the growing market for dental stools, by the end of the century dentists still had not articulated a practical justification for sitting down, reinforcing the view that this was a sociopolitical act, if not a salvo in a class war. An ad for the Practical Operating Stool, manufactured by Ransom & Randolph Co., of Toledo, Ohio, offered a sound rationale for apologists. In the 1911 Marshall Dental Mfg. Co. catalog, the copywriter addressed the benefits of sitting thusly:

Fatigue impairs a dentist's productiveness, his skill and his health. A tired man cannot do as well for his patients *or for himself* as he might if he had conserved his strength. The Practical Stool is a conserver of strength, and its continued *or occasional* use produce a restful feeling that is unknown to the man who works standing all day.

Once the argument was advanced that sitting could enhance productivity, it was inevitable that engineers interested in cold efficiency and precision would turn their attention to dental stool design. In 1922 the forerunner of the modern dental stool was unveiled in Germany. Key distinguishing features were a saddle seat and a revolutionary wheeled base the stool sat upon, allowing it to be rolled into position at lightning speed, no doubt depriving patients of any time to resist.

Many dentists, however, continued standing. It was only with the development of the modern contoured dental chair for their patients that all dentists took a seat.

Taking it Lying Down

AT THE 1962 World's Fair in Seattle, multitudes flocked to see the wonders of modern science and technology. A mock-up of a rocket ship provided a tangible artifact of the coming space age. But the sleek reclining chair on which the astronaut was to be seated was not designed for space travel. It was actually a Ritter-Euphorian Chair, made for use in a dental office. When it was unveiled in 1960, it won the Industrial Design Institute's Gold Medal Award as the first major change in dental chairs in fifty years. The evolution had been going on for far longer. Dr. Richard A. Glenner has led research into its history.

The first dental chairs were simply conventional armchairs. Pierre Fouchard, credited with first getting patients off the floor and into chairs, recommended one with armrests and a back high enough to support the patient's head. Early American dentist Josiah Flagg took an ordinary Windsor chair and fastened a headrest of his own design to it. James Snell made a chair with an adjustable seat and backrest in 1832. By the 1850s, a variety of commercially manufactured dentists chairs were available. More flexibility was invested in them. Some allowed the back to be tilted forward and back and were outfitted with adjustable headrests and footrests for the comfort of the patient's extremities.

Following the Civil War, dental chairs adopted a more utilitarian appearance. Wood was replaced by metal. Cushions replaced thick, padded upholstery. The quaint colonial look was relegated to the past, and with it some old-fashioned comfort. Favorites whose names resounded in parlors of the past, like Ask's Dental Chair and the Perkins, were banished to the rubbish heap, supplanted by models made by S. S. White, Morrison, and others. These featured reclining mechanisms allowing patients to be tipped backward easily. The S. S. White model, a stark, proto-alienlike design, remained popular for almost a century, up until the 1960s.

Yet from a developmental point of view, these models can be seen as mere evolutionary cul-de-sacs, for the antecedent of today's chair is a model introduced in 1883, the "Relax-Chair," designed exclusively for use with general anesthesia. It looked more like a chaise longue than a chair.

Little progress was made during the first half of the twentieth century. By the postwar years, most dentists had accepted the benefits of performing their ministrations while seated, and of having their patients in a reclining position. What was needed was a way to meld these two exigencies into a single piece of equipment that provided a chair for both dentist and patient.

In 1954, Dr. Sanford S. Golden, who had started his practice on a stool as an army dentist in 1942, convened a team of specialists in California to develop a reclining dental chair that could seat a dentist as well as the patient. Four years later the design was completed and the patents were turned over to the Ritter Co., a manufacturer of dental office equipment. The resulting production model was the Ritter-Euphorian Chair. The one-piece construction had no break in the back. According to Golden, this eliminated backaches. The distinctive contour became known as the Golden Curve. The sculpted look set a tone for futuristic, space-age modernity. Foot pedals controlled elevation and inclination—patients could be swung fifty degrees from the vertical—allowing the chair to be adjusted without any contamination of the hands.

Golden elaborated on his theories in an article, "Human Factors Applied to Study of Dentist and Patient in Dental Environment: a Static Appraisal," published in the *Journal of the American Dental Association*. The fifty-degree angle, he wrote, improved patient circulation and lessened fatigue, in addition to providing dentists with improved oral access. The impact of the article was immediate, leading to the widespread adoption of both reclining dental chairs and sitdown dentistry.

The Ritter-Euphorian was placed in several dental schools during its debut year. Trade advertisements stressed the comfort to patients and ease of oral access for dentists. Yet dentists seemed disinclined to take advantage of their Golden opportunity. The Euphorium design never achieved widespread commercial success. Its high cost was one factor, as was the one-piece design that was its hallmark. The design resulted in patient's legs being thrust farther skyward the more their backs were tilted horizontally. Dentists needed a chair with an articulated back and seat, independently motorized, capable of putting a patient in a true reclining position.

In 1958, John Naughton, founder of the Comfra Lounge Chair Company, manufacturers of vibrating chairs, had a fateful meeting with a pair of dentists at a dental convention. They challenged him to create a more comfortable dental chair. His first prototype test model was molded from a set of Tinkertoys. After what an executive of the Den-Tal-Ez Mfg. Co. later described as "many long hours of research and work," Naughton removed the arms and bottom attachment from an existing dental chair and created an articulating back.

Finally, Naughton's prototype chair was completed and placed in a dentist's office for evaluation. The dentist was impressed but Naughton was not satisfied. Unlike Golden's design, his had no seat for the dentist, and after observing the dentist and the chair in a clinical setting, Naughton was convinced the dentist should be working from the seated position. Some dentists were concerned that having patients lie supine could lead to debris from dental procedures falling down their throats, but Naughton demonstrated these concerns were unfounded.

His first production-model reclining dental chair, delivered in a beat-up $150 hearse, was operated by hand using hydraulic cylinders and a brake, which controlled the angle of recumbency. This was the progenitor of the chair that would take the place of honor in dental offices across the country. By the late 1960s, Naughton's recliner was the chair of choice among dentists. The chair most patients recline on today is based on the original Den-Tal-Ez model, now built by new manufacturers. And Naughton's original, hearse-delivered chair can be found (if one were to rummage around the basement) in the Smithsonian Institution.

Orifice Hours

DENTAL OFFICE DECOR was evolving in step with technological innovation and public taste. As dentistry became more involved with cosmetic procedures, concern about the appearance of the dental office itself grew. A connection between tasteful appointments and patients' appointments gained acceptance. The dentist's domain became a nexus of aesthetics and anesthetics. But the impact of interior design was not felt by patients alone. A 1924 manual, for example, "Practice Building Suggestions," recommended using mahogany for office woodwork.

> If a dentist is continually working under high tension, mahogany finishes would be most desirable for him, for the reason that mahogany in itself suggests quietness and would help to tone down the dentist. Oftentimes a nervous condition in the dentist can be traced to operating room cross lights playing on the improper wall treatment, and this effect is intensified in the light finishes of equipment used.

As the nascent "designer" product concept of the 1960s and 1970s found its way to dental offices, dentists engaged architects to create patient-friendly office environments and manufacturers came out with ever sleeker, less hostile-looking equipment. The growing design sophistication reached a zenith in 1970 when a dental office won the American Institute of Interior Design Award for the first time. Interestingly, this award-winning office featured a semiretro look: antique furnishings along with high-tech equipment. No doubt the mahogany-loving author of "Practice Building Suggestions" would have approved.

Time-management studies, the rage of corporate America in the 1950s, also found their way into dental offices. With the multiple tasks dentists performed, surely there was a way to make their operations more efficient. One ergonomics expert suggested dentists keep a motion study of their activities on a daily basis. They could then accurately assess the time they spent on various aspects of their business, from treatment to administration. The results enabled them to redesign the office, thereby saving steps and time. Dentists who followed these recommendations did indeed improve their offices' time-management performance. However, there were drawbacks to this approach. Although more "efficient," the application of time-management principles led to a lessening of physical activity of dentists and their assistants. The disturbing consequences became clear within a decade.

A 1963 study, "Body Mechanics Applied to the Practice of Dentistry" found that work habits of the "efficient" dentist, from a time and motion study point of view, were physically debilitating and could, over time, lead to illness and shorten one's career. Of course, then the dentist would have plenty of time on his hands, the one thing these studies always found a shortage of.

The Spin on Drills

THE WHINE OF the dental drill is extremely effective in provoking anxiety among dental phobics. The whizzing and whirring that rises and falls, clearly audible (if not somehow magically amplified) in waiting rooms, no doubt provokes a flood of brain chemicals among those affected, designed to assist flight from the area at maximum speed. Paradoxically, these individuals should be comforted by the dizzying drone. For the introduction of high-speed, or ultraspeed drills in the 1950s was one of the major advances of the modern era, greatly facilitating treatment of the teeth.

Jewelers bow drills were the first drilling instruments used to prepare cavities for filling. Being rigid, they proved poorly adapted to the dark contours of the mouth. The first practical advance in dental drilling technology was the coiled spring wire and flexible shaft, introduced in 1829 by a Scottish engineer. This was the inspiration for the first flexible cable hand drill, introduced by Charles Merry of St. Louis in 1858. These drills were manually powered—actually foot-powered, leaving the dentist's hands free while the foot pumped up the power.

The first motor-driven dental engine was patented in England in 1864, driven by a key-wound spring motor. However it was weak and inefficient, and foot engines remained more popular. When George F. Green created an electrically driven dental engine in 1870, it signaled the end of manual drills, and a milestone in the electrification of the dental office.

Industrial drill users availed themselves to high-speed technology long before dentists. Dental drills spun at the relatively slow rotation rates of 1,000 to 2,000 rpm. Before the mid-1940s, 4,000 rpm appears to be the top speed any dentists used. Higher speeds, it was feared, would make the hand drills harder to control. But a discovery made during a project conducted for the Australian Air Force by dentist John Walsh in 1949 helped to change conventional thinking. Walsh found that higher rotational speeds "produced vibrational frequencies that were more acceptable to patients than those produced at conventional speeds."

Walsh had first considered the relation between drill speed and discomfort in 1945. Most dentists knew that the sound conductivity of teeth and bone was a major factor in the unpleasantness of the dental drill. Walsh used tuning forks to test this connection by experimenting with a drill on his own teeth. He found the vibrations at just over middle C, 256 Hz, were the most unpleasant, while those two octaves higher and above ceased to be perceived as vibrations at all. It was this observation that led him to begin developing a high speed drill.

Work was also underway in the United States. In 1953, a team led by Dr. Robert J. Nelson at the National Bureau of Standards, in a project funded by the ADA, created a hydraulically powered turbine that achieved a speed of 61,000 rpm. It used a high-pressured stream of fluid to drive the drill. This was the first clinically operating turbine dental drill. (Turbine drills had been seen as early as the 1880s, but the inadequacy of the ball bearings and fears of what would happen if they broke in a patient's mouth were among the concerns that kept them out of dentists' hands.)

From that point on, it became a race for speed. The following year the air-turbine handpiece was introduced. By the end of the decade a drill capable of reaching an ultraspeed of 1,000,000 rpm had been demonstrated. Meanwhile, many older model drills in dental offices around the country were being souped up and retrofitted with better motors capable of faster spin rates. Disconnecting the resistors, cleaning the engine armature, and eliminating the slack in the belt drive alone could boost the speed of these units to 12,000 rpm.

Today, turbine handpiece dental drills, with their air bearings, typically spin at over 400,000 rpm. The sound may be annoying, but the actual discomfort their contact causes with the benumbed tooth is virtually nil. The speed allows the bur to cut through the enamel and dentine quickly and accurately. At least, that's the spin any dentist would like to put on this subject.

Soon even these turbine drills may be no more than quaint curiosities of a bygone era. In 1997 the United States Food and Drug Administration approved the first laser dental "drill." During testing on more than 1,300 teeth, only three patients requested local anesthetic. The laser burns through the decay without affecting undamaged parts of the tooth. There is no pressure and no vibration. However, initially eye goggles were mandated for dentists and patients to protect their eyes from the intense laser beam.

From Oral to Aural

THAT TEETH ARE sensitive to vibrations had been noted long before dentists began drilling into them. This sensitivity stimulated some bold thinkers to consider ways in which the teeth could be used for hearing.

Hieronymus Cardanus, a physician, mathematician, and jurist from Pavia, first proposed using the teeth for auditory reception in 1550 in his book, *De subtilitate*. Sound, he stated, could be conducted to brain's auditory center by biting on a stick of hard wood. Half a century later, Capivaccio attempted to find a rational justification for Cardanus's speculation. He described it in terms of mechanical action, tracing the sound's path from the wood, through the teeth, to the cranial bones, and thence brainward. Beethoven, after losing his hearing, was known to employ a method similar to this when he tried out his compositions on the piano, using a ruler instead of a stick. And though his ears may have failed him, his dentition didn't. Beethoven was said to have "a fine mouth, dazzling teeth, and powerful jaws that grind nuts."

In 1789 an "audiophone" was introduced, constructed from a flexible Japanese hand fan, curved in such a way that it conveniently fit between the teeth. But efforts to harness the teeth as ears reached the apogee of their low orbit in the twentieth century, when a United States patent was granted to the Dentiphone in 1928. It used a metal rod to transmit sound captured by a trumpetlike tube, to the teeth. With the introduction of electroacoustic sound transmission, the teeth were abandoned in favor of other auditory routes to the hearing centers.

Toothpick Tales

PEOPLE WERE JABBING sticks of wood between their teeth long before Cardanus, though for cleaning, rather than hearing. Signs of toothpick use have been seen in Neanderthal skulls. A contemporary anthropologist claims "As far as can be empirically documented, the oldest demonstrable human habit is picking one's teeth."

Today the venerable wooden toothpick is endangered by the plastic variety. While it still enjoys supremacy, let us pay homage to the rich history of teeth-picking, and the implements used for this purpose through recorded time.

Toothpicks were popular across ancient Asia, India, and the Middle East, made from sharpened fibrous sticks, or from quill, bronze, iron, silver, or gold. References to wooden toothpicks (as well as mouthwashes) are found in the old Hebrew Talmud, and in Greek and Roman writings. The Greeks used blades of straw, reeds, or a quill to clean the teeth. Agathocles, the despotic ruler of Syracuse, was assassinated by a toothpick in 289 B.C.; it had been soaked in poison.

Romans, placing a premium on oral hygiene, regarded toothpicks among the necessities in the toilets of ladies of fashion. Martial (Marcus Valerius Martiales) (A.D. ca. 40–ca. 103) wrote they were generally of lentisk wood (also called the toothpick tree), though more precious materials were no doubt also used. Pliny denounced using vulture quills to clean the teeth, as it resulted in foul breath. He recommended the quill of a porcupine, instead.

The Muslim prophet Mohammed favored toothpicks carved from aromatic aloe wood dipped into the fountain of holy water at Mecca. He was so enamored of the habit that he appointed a "master of the toothpick," who carried the device behind his ear. The Koran itself states, "a prayer which is preceded by the use of a toothpick is worth seventy-five ordinary prayers" and "you shall clean your mouth for this is a means of praising God."

The Parsi, a group that migrated to India from Persia between the eighth and tenth centuries, are believed to have elevated toothpick use to a religious rite of sorts, and the Gonds, another almost forgotten civilization, were known to bury the dead with their toothpicks.

Little is known of toothpick use in the West after the fall of Rome until the Middle Ages, when toothpicks regained their positions of prominence. In France during the Renaissance, toothpicks could be found stuck in desserts as well as proffered along with a plate and napkin at each place setting. They took on all the ornamentation and trappings of other personal luxury products of the time. Made of gold, silver, or ivory, they were sometimes set with precious jewels and inlaid with gems. Some were worn on chains around the neck. Picking the teeth was an upper-class trait, lower classes being unable to afford toothpicks.

Soon proper use of the toothpick became a matter of etiquette. *The Tanhausers Court Manners*, published in Innsbruck in 1393, advised readers that picking one's teeth during a meal was as rude as "sneezing and snarfeling into your hand while eating at table."

They were even considered important dowry items. When the infanta Louise Marie Therese of Parma wed a prince of Asturias, a dozen valuable toothpicks were part of the package. They were not necessarily community property. In Saxony, for example, a woman's toothpick remained her property, though the vessel it came in—a gem-encrusted cask, say—was not. And lest the value and ornamentation of the items ever detract from their purpose, a 1716 book of manners reminded ladies that they were nothing more than the silver tools "with which the wench, when something comes between her teeth during eating, can free such particles."

Medicinal use was likewise recommended. In the late 1400s Joannes Arculanus championed using thin strips of wood, especially bitter or styptic varieties, such as aloes or pine, to remove food and avoid cavities.

England was not immune to the pull of the pick. On June 27, 1488, James IV of Scotland bought "twa tuthpikis of gold with a chenze"— two gold toothpicks with a chain. His son, James V, ordered "Ane pennare of silver to keip pyke teeth in"—silver case worn at the midriff for holding toothpicks.

Shakespeare's canon, which contains several allusions to toothpick use, underscores the class difference it reflected and reinforced in his verse: "He seems to be more noble in being fantastical: a great man, I'll warrant; I know by the picking one's teeth."

Naturally, some of the less couth imitated the highbrows, using whatever utensil was available. A knife was often the instrument of choice by default. This was considered poor manners, as an instructional poem of the late 1500s indicates:

> *Pick not they teeth with they knyfe*
> *Nor with they fyngers ende,*
> *But take a stick, or some cleane thyng,*
> *Then doe you not offende.*
> Rhodes, 1577

Fauchard was not impressed with the popular high-fashion designs. He condemned metal toothpicks as being injurious to the mouth, with copper or iron causing the most damage.

In the 1800s, toothpicks remained out of the reach of most consumers, even as new technologies were roiling old markets. For example, Monsieur Bardin of Joinville-le-Pont, near Paris, found the invention of the steel pen had ruined the market for the quills from his two million geese. Quickly altering production, he created a quill toothpick, instead, which became one of the first mass-market toothpicks.

Today, Fauchard would be happy to see a sense of sanity has returned to this ancient habit. Now, most people in the civilized world pick their teeth with cheap, effective, and simple wooden toothpicks. The great majority come from the town of Strong, Maine, self-proclaimed "Toothpick Capital of the World" and home of the biggest toothpick factory in the United States. Writer Sue Hubbell picked through historical records to find out how Strong came to claim its title.

Charles Forster, a Bostonian, was on business in Brazil in the mid-1800s when he saw large, hand-whittled toothpicks from Portugal being sold in big boxes as disposable appliances. He bought some and sent them to his wife in Boston, who shared them with guests. The reception must have been positive, for when Forster returned to Boston in 1865, he went to work for a wooden shoe-peg manufacturer and began experimenting with equipment in the factory, trying to develop a machine that could cut toothpicks. By 1869 he'd achieved success. The machine he invented could make as many toothpicks in a minute as a hand-whittler could make in a day. Today's toothpick-making machines are little changed from Forster's original concept.

Forster found white birch as the wood of choice, which he found in abundance in Maine. Yet the world did not beat a path to his door. Boston restaurant owners ignored his product. "They didn't think that proper Bostonians would want to sit around after dinner picking their teeth with a slender piece of wood," he lamented.

The turnaround came at Boston's Union Oyster House, an establishment still in business today. Forster had recruited some Harvard scholars with the promise of a free meal if they'd help him in his plan to sell toothpicks. The plan, as Forster outlined it later:

> After dinner, the Harvard student, in a loud voice, was supposed to ask his waiter for a toothpick. If the restaurant didn't have any, then the young man was supposed to complain loudly, and inform the waiter that he would never again eat in the establishment.

After five or six Harvard men had stormed out following their well-rehearsed display, the Oyster House started buying Forster's toothpicks. Forster moved his toothpick factory to Maine a few years later to be closer to his raw material. Ownership has long since changed hands, but even today the building at the Strong, Maine, plant bears the name Forster's, Inc. Today the machines are computer-driven, and highly automated. It takes only a couple of hours to turn a birch log into boxes of toothpicks. The factory's ten or so employees turn out about 20 million toothpicks a day. On that same day, toothpicks will cause an average twenty-four accidents, according to the Consumer Products Safety Commission.

The Big Brush Off

LIKE THE TOOTHPICK, the toothbrush is in a state of transition. Manually powered brushes are joined by an ever-widening array of electrified models. But compared to its slender cousin the pick, the toothbrush is a recent innovation. In their place, the ancients devised a variety of teethcleansing tools.

Hippocrates recommended using a small ball of wool moistened in honey, and then a rinse of dill, aniseed, myrrh, and white wine. Pliny reported that dentifrices were made from the ashes of dogs' teeth mixed with honey, and from pumice.

In India, Susruta Samhita, author of the basic text of Indian medicine, advised that "One should rise early in the morning and brush ones teeth. The tooth brush should consist of a fresh twig of a tree free from any knots, 12 fingers in length, and as thick as one's small finger." He also recommended daily use of a cleansing paste made from honey, oil, and other ingredients.

Fresh sticks of the bead tree *(melia azedarach)* and mango *(mangiferra indica)* were often used for teethcleaning implements, as was wood from arak, *salvadora persica,* often known as the toothbrush tree.

The toothbrush appeared in Europe late in the middle ages. They may have first appeared in France. In a 1649 letter to Sir Ralph Verney, an English friend asks him to inquire in Paris for the "little brushes for making cleane of the teeth, most covered with sylver and some few with gold and sylver twiste, together with some petits bouettes to put them in."

They were slow to catch on. More than a century later, in 1755, Samuel Johnson made no mention of toothbrushes in his dictionary. He did, however, refer to a toothpick and a toothpicker. Cloths and sponges were the primary tools for cleaning teeth. Toothbrushes remained a rare luxury until after 1850, when manufacturing created a large, affordable supply, bringing them into widespread use.

However, just as neglect of oral care had its risks, so too did some toothbrushes. An Albany, New York, surgeon performing an appendectomy found the patient's disorder was due to the presence of an accumulation of toothbrush bristles.

"Cheap toothbrushes," remarked the doctor, "are responsible for many obscure throat, stomach, and intestinal ailments. The bristles are only glued on, and come off by the half-dozen when wet and brought in contact with the teeth."

The toothpaste we think of as inextricably linked to the toothbrush only began to replace tooth powders and tinctures in the late 1800s. It caught on as a popular form of dentifrice after it was packed in collapsible metal tubes like artists' paints, which had been packaged that way for many years. The pastes were hawked with all the imagination and hucksterism of their powdered predecessors.

Pebeco toothpaste was marketed through a campaign of fears, warning that the lack of exercise the mouth glands received from the "soft foods of the modern diet," could lead to tooth decay. Wrigley's Gum encouraged consumers to take after chorus girls, who kept fit "in all respects," avoiding "flabby face lines" by chewing Wrigley's Spearmint Gum for exercise.

Custer's Last Toothbrush

CAN A SINGLE toothbrush tell us as much about its owner as about evolving oral health-care habits? If a case can be made in the affirmative, one compelling piece of evidence would be Custer's Last Toothbrush.

When General George Armstrong Custer set out for his fateful encounter at the Little Bighorn, he left behind his toothbrush, a model made by Caswell, Hazard & Co. Had he brought it along, the opportunity to speculate on the connection between the general's personality and his personal toothbrush might have been lost forever. Today it is on view at the Little Bighorn Battlefield National Monument. The toothbrush appears well suited to the egotistical, outspoken general; the large size looks like it was made for a big mouth. It sports fifteen bushy rows of bristles, compared to today's standard dozen. And the bristles look none the worse for wear, perhaps helping corroborate Custer's foul-mouthed reputation.

Military historians will doubtless continue to debate what could have been done to save the Seventh Cavalry from the Sioux, Cheyenne, and their allies that day. But subsequent studies of the teeth of some of the soldiers who died with Custer on June 25, 1876, reveal little could have been done to save them from future dental problems. Abscesses, caries, periodontitis, attrition, antemortem tooth loss, and indications of tobacco use were found among an octet of dental remains examined.

Dental historians and psychobiographers can only wonder if these soldiers' brush with destiny would have ended differently had their commander favored a different brush himself. As for the general, we can now add an important character insight to the legacy history has already accorded him: He died with his boots on, and his toothbrush far off.

Root Canal: Pulp Facts

ROOT CANAL: PERHAPS no two words in dentistry equal their power to terrify. Why is this so? Why should drilling through healthy, white enamel, boring into quivering, abscessed, and acutely sensitive pulp, then eviscerating the nerve-filled root before cleaning its narrowest passageways with sharp needles, so bother those to whom it is done? In a time when the procedure is essentially painless, one must search the mind as well as the mouth for possible answers. We, however, will confine ourselves to the oral cavity.

Root canal, today performed by endodontists, signifies removing the pulp and nerves of an abscessed tooth and filling the excavation. Pinpointing when such pulp treatments were first done is difficult. An 1831 text by London dentist James Snell discussed the application of silver nitrate to what he called "ulcerated surface," or exposed pulp, protected by a temporary plug of mastic. This appears to be the first written record of treating the pulp of teeth, though his account makes the practice sound common to the era. Records from the United States indicate American dentists of the time were also familiar with pulp procedures.

The pain must have been unimaginable by present standards. Shearjashub Spooner suggested using arsenic trioxide to devitalize the pulp in 1836, the first successful method of controlling pain incident to pulp extirpation. Many practitioners condemned the practice, owing to the destruction wrought on surrounding tissue, but arsenic soon became the dentist's agent of choice for desensitizing dentin and devitalizing pulp. Now that the root had been rendered painless, a slew of "ingenious" instruments were developed, allowing dentists to scoop out pulp and dredge the canals, with euphonious names like the barbed nerve broach. With the introduction of the improved anesthetics and instruments of the twentieth century, the procedure became essentially painless.

Despite the lack of tangible sensations the therapy produces, root canal now occupies the position with which extractions were formerly honored, the apotheosis of painful dental procedures. This evolution can be seen in the two cinematic versions of *The Little Shop of Horrors*, the story of a toothsome, human-eating plant. In the original production, directed by Roger Corman, the masochistic patient (portrayed by Jack Nicholson) came to the dental office asking to have all his teeth pulled. In the remake, the masochist (Bill Murray) begged the dentist (Steve Martin) to give him a root canal.

10

The Million-Dollar Smile

Dentistry, Hollywood, and Oral Image-Making

L ET US RISE FROM OUR RECUMBENT POSITION ON THE DENTIST'S contoured recliner for a moment and look at teeth not in the direct illumination of the dental examining light, but in the warm glow of contemporary society's preoccupation with appearance, self-improvement, and self-deception. Here, beyond the clinical surroundings, dentition has come full circle. Focus has returned to glorification of the tooth. Their totemic power to suggest, if not bestow vigor and vitality has been restored. Here they are not signs of a crumbling infrastructure, of moral and social decay, but again symbols of power and glamour, and the mouth itself, the ultimate consumer accessory.

As a body part, the mouth is one of the progenitors of the self-improvement movement. The public was spending vast sums on crowns (in lay terms, "caps") and braces before anyone ever heard of ab flexors, health clubs, or liposuction.

The modern era of tooth veneration was born of postwar prosperity and optimism. The free world had much to smile about, and everyone wanted a smile as bright, straight, and uniform as a row of identical suburban homes. Owning that dream mouth was suddenly affordable. As swords were beaten into dental drills, dentists became agents of assimilation. Even as the fight against tooth decay escalated, waged by a public energized by toothpaste commercials and sublimated Cold War fears, dentistry devoted more attention to cosmetic concerns.

But an ambivalence was at work, one whose antecedents we have seen in antiquity. Even with pain banished, the patient's relationship with the dentist remained unsettled, a confusing blend of gratitude and antipathy. Let us examine the rich historical residue of these conflicted emotions.

Unsightly Film

HOLLYWOOD CAN CLAIM title as the uncrowned capital of cosmetic dentistry, thanks to the demands of the film industry. Stars required perfect teeth and dentists were essential for realizing the illusion Hollywood strove to create. Even child star Shirley Temple had her teeth capped to enhance her photogenicity. Years later she described how she lost her two front caps after sneezing, shutting down production on a film until the caps could be replaced.

Perhaps the film community resented this dental dependency. How else to explain the legacy of unsightly film that Hollywood left on dental work, or its habit of denigrating dentists onscreen?

Tinseltown auteurs could make little claim for originality in this department. Visual artists had turned their attention on dental practices centuries before Hollywood's heyday, often portraying its practitioners in a less than flattering light. When art turned its attention to dentistry, typically it was the dentist, not the artist who suffered. Today these paintings serve as historical records documenting how protodentists conducted their trade. We can only hope future historians don't employ Hollywood films, or the work of early photographers, in the same manner.

As the art and science of photography developed in the mid-nineteenth century, the lens of the new invention was turned on the dental parlor. Staged comic scenes were especially popular, portraying dentists in the most sadistic and incompetent light. They were pictured, for example using heavy tools and brutal methods to perform dental procedures on terrorized patients. Others were shown employing bizarre gadgets in scenes satirizing the day's obsession with electrical therapy devices recommended for toothaches and other maladies. The photos were often created in stereoviews made for enjoyment as home entertainment, much like today's television.

Dentists were also the frequent butt of vaudeville comedy. In the early days of moving pictures, these comic routines were often recreated for film. The popularity of films doomed vaudeville and also brought down the curtain on the live street performances and traveling dental and medicine shows of the late nineteenth century. But the new medium proved more than capable of taking up where vaudeville comedians left off.

Mouth Parts

THE EARLIEST FILM in which dentistry played at least a supporting role was 1902s *At Last! That Awful Tooth,* directed by George Albert Smith. Apparently the film was little more than a deadpan examination of the title subject, prefiguring the directorial style that would earn Andy Warhol acclaim with films such as *Empire State* and *Sleep* over half a century later.

Early screen goddess Mary Pickford appeared in *The Fair Dentist* in 1911. A still from the film, showing the eighteen-year-old star extracting a tooth, is all that remains of the production, and this scene may have actually been lifted from a forgotten Pickford flick of the era. A decade later, Pickford extracted her own tooth in *Little Lord Fauntleroy* (1921), using the old tooth-tied-to-the-door-knob routine.

Meanwhile, respectable dentists sought to use the new medium to elevate their profession. By 1913, the Mouth Hygiene Association had produced an eighteen-minute silent film, *Toothache.* Directed by Dr. W. G. Eversole, the one-reel movie was produced in Indianapolis by the Motionscope Company on a budget of about $500 and distributed to dentists and dental organizations in twenty states and some nine foreign countries. *Your Mouth: A Standardized Educational Motion Picture of the Care and Use of the Human Mouth* was released nationally in 1922. The one-reeler was created with the input of over 100 specialists by dentist-director Edwin N. Kent.

In December of that same year, Kansas City dentist Thomas B. McCrum inked a down-on-his-luck twenty-one-year-old filmmaker to create a children's film on dental health. Dr. McCrum had to come to the filmmaker's office—the Laugh-o-Gram Studio—to sign the contract because the young man had no shoes. His only pair was in the shoe shop getting fixed and he couldn't afford the $1.50 to reclaim them.

The contract to produce and make 500 copies of the film rescued the young filmmaker, Walt Disney, from poverty, providing the funds to get his new company off the ground. The resulting production, *Tommy Tucker's Tooth,* a silent, fifteen-minute live-action film with animated inserts, focused on the fastidious young Tommy Tucker and a hygienically challenged contemporary, Jimmy Jones. When Tommy is hired for the job both youngsters apply for, Jimmy realizes the error of his ways, cleans up his mouth and his act, and eventually finds gainful employment. Disney went on to make more educational films for the dental market for thirty years, as well as produce a variety of mass-market entertainments.

Despite these noble efforts to harness its educational powers, cinema would prove a painful medium for oral health-care providers.

What is thought to be the first commercial movie to deal with the subject of dental visits is *Laughing Gas* in 1914. Written, starring, and directed by Charlie Chaplin, the Tramp portrays a dental assistant to Dr. Pain, who takes charge of the office and runs amuck, ultimately grabbing the nose of a pretty young patient in his forceps and kissing her. It set the tone for most celluloid treatments of dentistry that followed. Harold Lloyd, Buster Keaton, Red Skelton, Abbot and Costello, and Jerry Lewis were among the comedians who would eventually use their mocking humor to demean the profession.

Legendary film figure Hal Roach released *The Dippy Dentist* in 1919. Though it covered similar ground to Chaplin's, this is still a historically important film, as it was shot on location in an early urban dental office. Thus, it gives an accurate view of equipment and parlors of the era. Indeed, although their portrayal of dentists is far from accurate, early dental comedies have proven valuable in charting the evolution of their offices, from simple rooms without plumbing or electricity to the antiseptic and electrified offices of the 1920s.

Laurel and Hardy delivered their first dental defamation in 1928's *Leave 'Em Laughing*. It opens with Laurel awaking with a toothache late at night, and ends following many painful pratfalls with the pair wandering the streets, dazed from laughing gas, after Hardy's tooth has been mistakenly extracted instead of Laurel's. Obviously the performances struck a nerve with audiences, for Laurel and Hardy's first all-talking movie, *Pardon Us*, featured a dentist's skit.

During the 1930s, the screen's ritual ridicule reached its apotheosis with *The Dentist*, written by and starring W. C. Fields. A twenty-minute short, this was Field's only role in which he created a completely unsympathetic protagonist, a character exhibiting a total lack of compassion and consideration along with an excess of cruelty and licentious liberty.

The Three Stooges made a trio of films with dental bits: *All the World's A Stooge* (1941), *I Can Hardly Wait* (1943), and *The Tooth Will Out* (1951). In the first, the three portrayed window-washers-turned-dentists. The second borrows heavily from the work of Laurel and Hardy's filmed dental misadventures. The Stooges' slapstick routines and physical comedy could themselves be dentally dangerous—Stooge Larry Fine had a tooth knocked out in the filming of one of their productions.

Even Tinseltown tough guy Jimmy Cagney and Hollywood he-man Gary Cooper got in the act. Both starred in versions of a dental drama that found its way onto screen in three different productions over the span of a decade and a half. It was originally released as *One Sunday Afternoon* in 1933, starring Gary Cooper and Fay Wray. Cagney's performance, seen when the story reappeared as *The Strawberry Blond* in 1941, is considered definitive. Set at the turn of the century, Cagney portrays a graduate of a dental correspondence school who loses Rita Hayworth to a shady construction contractor. At the end of the last reel, when the contractor shows up for emergency dental work, Cagney plans to kill him with an overdose of laughing gas, but at the last minute relents, and merely performs the extraction without anesthesia. The story returned under the same title in 1948, this time as a musical.

Writer-director Preston Sturges looked toward the oral cavity for inspiration in *The Greatest Moment* (1944), adapted from *Triumph Over Pain*, the story of Dr. William T. G. Morton, the discredited claimant to the honor of anesthesia's inventor. The film has been labeled as "the beginning of its director's decline."

The wide-open spaces of the American West and the American mouth met in *Texas*, a 1941 film starring William Holden and Glenn Ford. The movie featured Edgar Buchanan as a frontier dentist, ready to check teeth for decay anytime—even in the midst of a gunfight. It was an apt piece of typecasting: Buchanan was a dentist turned actor. He went on to costar in the TV series *Petticoat Junction*.

A more noteworthy treatment of the frontier dentist was offered by Bob Hope in 1948's *Paleface*. Set in the 1870s, Hope portrays Painless Peter Potter (acknowledged as a takeoff on the early twentieth-century dental gadfly Painless Parker), exiled to an itinerant life by his incompetence. Joined in a marriage of convenience (hers) to Calamity Jane (Jane Russell), who is secretly working for the government, the inept dentist is duped into believing he is responsible for the straight-shooting heroics Calamity actually performs. Recognizing the carnal patina Hollywood at times applied to the practice of dentistry, can we ignore this film's sexual subtext? The impotent, frustrated filler of cavities paired with the gun-slinging, predatory, and sexually charged woman of the West: Who will drill whom first?

Audiences came back for a checkup when the sequel, *Son of Paleface*, was released in 1952, now featuring Roy Rogers and Douglas Dumbrille. Finally, a pale remake of the original brought Don Knotts to the title role as a bumbling Philadelphia dentist in *The Shakiest Gun in the West*, released in 1968.

After decades of lighthearted digs at dentists, Hollywood took off the surgical gloves in 1976, presenting a chilling portrait of the dentist as sadistic torturer in the *The Marathon Man*. If that wasn't enough to get audiences riled at the profession, the dentist was personified by none other than Auschwitz Angel of Death, Dr. Joseph Mengele (Laurence Olivier). The camera pays close attention to Olivier's use of a drill and a healthy, unanesthetized tooth nerve to extract information from Dustin Hoffman.

The dentist as lecher, first seen in Charlie Chaplin's *Laughing Gas*, received a reworking in the mid-1980s in *Compromising Positions*. Clearly, dentists' dalliances were no longer viewed with such a tolerant eye: The movie's overly amorous dentist, portrayed by Joe Mantegna, is murdered.

The musical version of *Little Shop of Horrors*, released in 1986, tried to restore some of the fun and broad-humored innocence to the dental flick. Based on the successful Broadway musical, adapted from the original Roger Corman exploitation film of 1961, it gave comedian Steve Martin the opportunity to put his own comic spin on the dentistry. "I'm your dentist," the star sings, "I get high on the pain I inflict, I thrill when I drill a bicuspid, although it may cause my patients distress."

Yet it is clear who has been most pained and distressed by these negative representations: dentists themselves. As one writer noted, "the dentist who can bear to watch these films at all, must learn to accept them as an occupational hazard that reduces his feeling of self-worth."

Given the plethora of negative representations and resulting perceptions, dentists cannot be blamed for wanting to tell their side of the story. In the early 1980s, the American Dental Association planned a national pro-dentistry promotional effort. The centerpiece of the plan was an advertising campaign called the "Sparkle, Dazzle, Glow" series, slated to run on TV and in magazines. The campaign's tag line was, "Dazzle. When your teeth have it, you have it. Go get some at your dentist's!" The initial TV commercial featured a smiling female patient, who was asked, "Where did you get that glow?" Her answer: "I get it at my dentist's regularly." Apparently the exchange was felt to be too sexually suggestive, and the plug was pulled on the entire campaign before a single commercial aired.

An Epic Dental Story

DESPITE THE LIGHTHEARTED condescension of mainstream moviemakers, dentistry and artistry came together in what critics have called one of the greatest productions in Hollywood history, *Greed,* an epic silent film directed by Eric von Stroheim. This, the first noncomedy, feature-length movie about dentistry, was adapted from *McTeague: A Story of San Francisco,* an 1899 blockbuster by twenty-three-year-old Frank Norris. The story's protagonist, McTeague, was a violent, bitter brute of a dentist who kills his avaricious wife and her lover in a murderous rage. While fleeing justice, McTeague dies of thirst in the desert, handcuffed to the body of his last murder victim.

Von Stroheim, one of Hollywood's most tyrannical and overbearing directors, said it was his discovery of the book when he arrived destitute in the United States that inspired him to become a filmmaker. Through this story he attempted to achieve his artistic goal of "breaking through social hypocrisy and reasserting the corporeality of experience."

Originally nine-and-one-half hours long and taking up forty-two reels, *Greed* featured an all-star cast including Zazu Pitts and cost $470,000 to film, an unheard of sum for the time. Gold, so central to the dentist's trade, became the film's central visual metaphor, from the huge gilded tooth McTeague is movingly portrayed unpacking as he prepares to hang up the calling symbol outside his office, to the gleaming gold crown his wife displays when she opens her mouth. All the gold items in the black-and-white film were hand-tinted, frame by frame, a process that took several months.

The movie also contained the cinema's first scene in which a dentist is portrayed as a sexual predator (Chaplin's earlier stolen screen kiss notwithstanding), taking liberties with an anesthetized patient. The caption for this scene read, ". . . and she was absolutely without defense. Suddenly the animal in the man stirred and woke . . . it was a crisis . . . for which he was totally unprepared. Blindly . . . McTeague fought against it . . . but as he drew near to her again, the charm of her innocence and helplessness came over him afresh. It was a final protest against his resolution."

The movie premiered in December of 1924, though the length made viewing difficult. Dentists were greatly disturbed by the seduction scene, but as film critic Herman Weinberg saw it, *Greed* eloquently presented "what the frenzy for money, what the despair in losing it, could lead to, in any clime, at any time, and in any milieu."

A box-office disappointment, it was subsequently cut to less than two-and-a-half hours and released to the public. Stroheim refused to see the expurgated version. "I consider I have made only one real picture in my life and nobody ever saw that," he later said. "The poor, mangled, mutilated remains were shown as *Greed*. The man who cut my film had nothing on his mind but a hat."

In an interesting coda, *McTeague* reappeared as an opera, debuting at Chicago's Lyric Opera in 1992, with the bedeviled dentist's inner fury unleashed in melody as well as murder.

The Toothache Scarf

THE MOST COMMON image of toothache sufferers is likewise one of ridicule rather than compassion. Typically they are presented as objects of amusement, bandage-swaddled sad sacks, their swollen jaws protected by cloths wrapped around their heads. Here again modern image makers can claim no originality. This depiction hearkens back to a custom thousands of years old. Archeological records indicate Babylonians sometimes recited their incantations seeking relief from toothworms while wearing such bandages around their heads. The purpose of this dressing is unknown—perhaps to ward off spirits, hold a poultice in place, or keep the cheek warm, dental historians have suggested.

This was the first appearance of what is now labeled as a "toothache scarf," soft fabric applied to the cheek over the site of discomfort, often strapped in place by means of ligature or bandanna encircling the head. The Talmud recommends a scarflike bandage for toothaches, as well. The scarf was kept alive in Roman times. Their toothache remedies included linen cloths or rags applied to the cheek. Aulus Cornelius Celsus called for the head to be so wrapped after applying toothache medication to the jaw.

In *The Description of Instruments, Machines and Furniture Collected for Surgical and Medical Practice*, published in Florence in 1776, Father Don Ipolito Ferrarese reproduced a picture of the bust of a Roman soldier with a double rope bandage similar to a toothache scarf. This, however, was for supporting a fractured mandible rather than alleviating a toothache, so never mind. Some historians have suggested the toothache scarf is adapted from the "wimple" cloth, part of the uniform of some European nuns, an accessory that framed their faces and was arranged in folds beneath their chins, but this appears unlikely.

We can find the image of scarf-clad sufferers in the Italian medical manuscript of Ruggero de Frugardo, a treatise dating to the twelfth or thirteenth century, and in cartoons illustrating this same pained group from the eighteenth to the present. The French used handkerchiefs in a similar fashion, said to be folded "obliquely" and tied to the head, stuffed with a big piece of cotton. Of course, being French, the handkerchiefs were also often seasoned with condiments, including marjoram, potatoes, or perhaps "lukewarm cow dung."

A Verse to Pain

NOT ONLY VISUAL artists have made dentistry and teeth their subjects. Writers and poets have also left us indelible images of teeth. Greek dramatist Aristophanes went on record avowing to the uselessness of white teeth in the absence of anything to chew on. The subject entered the world of verse in earnest during Roman times. In one of this epigrams, Martial (A.D. ca. 40–ca. 103) mentioned one Cascellius, who "has grown rich as a senator among the fine ladies, and he cures tooth diseases," earning Cascellius the honor as the first dentist named in recorded history.

Martial was also the first to mention artificial teeth, baring his own fangs in his biting satire and establishing a tradition of what could be called literary criticism of these appliances.

Scotland's immortal Robert Burns (1759–1796) didn't mock teeth, but rather paid homage to their painful power in his "Address to the Toothache":

> *My curse upon the venom'd stang,*
> *That shoots my tortured gums alang;*
> *And throughout my lungs gies monie a twant,*
> *With gnawing vengeance,*
> *Tearing my nerves with bitter pang,*
> *Like racking engines.*

Not all cursed the dark toothache cavity. Some cajoled, as did John Heath-Stubbs in his entreaty, "A Charm Against the Toothache":

> *Venerable Mother Toothache*
> *Climb down from the white embattlement,*
> *Stop twisting in your yellow fingers*
> *The fourfold rope of nerves;*
> *And tomorrow I will give you a tot of whisky*
> *To hold in your cupped hands,*
> *A garland of anise-flowers,*
> *And three cloves like nails.*
> *And tell the attendant gnomes*
> *It is time to knock off now,*
> *To shoulder their little pickaxes,*
> *Their cold-chisels and drills.*
> *And you may mount by a silver ladder*
> *Into the sky, to grind*
> *In the cracked polished mortar*
> *Of the hollow moon.*

Perhaps nowhere in verse did artistry and dentistry combine to worse effect than in the epic poems of American dentist Solyman Brown (1790–1876). This excerpt from "The Dentologia—A poem on the Disease of the Teeth," found in the anthology *Very Bad Poetry*, gives a small indication of his excruciating handiwork:

. . . her lips disclosed to view,
Those ruined arches, veiled in ebon hue,
Where love had thought to feast the ravished sight
On orient gems reflecting snowy light,
Hope, disappointed, silently retired
Disgust triumphant came, and love expired! . . .

Whene'er along the ivory disks, are seen,
The filthy footsteps of the dark gangrene;
When caries come, with stealthy pace to throw
Corrosive ink spots on those banks of snow—
Brook no delay, ye trembling, suffering fair,
But fly for refuge to the dentist's care.

Shed-Tooth Rituals and the Tooth Fairy

GIVEN THE DEARNESS in which teeth are held and their role in projecting an image of power, the extraordinary efforts undertaken to preserve them is not surprising. Yet the loss of individual teeth has long been celebrated in cultures around the world. These shed-tooth rituals of ceremonies and prayers mark the loss of primary, deciduous, or "baby" teeth, a rite of passage signifying an important childhood transition.

Deciduous teeth have also been called "milk teeth," as they were thought to grow from mother's milk touching infants' gums while nursing. Evidence to the contrary could be dealt with harshly. The rare child born with erupted teeth was sometimes killed as a demon.

Known as "natal teeth" or "precocious teeth," erupted teeth are present in about one in 3,000 live births. Lower incisors are the teeth most usually seen. These dentally precocious babies have drawn attention throughout history. Pliny noted two such examples, one of whom who subsequently went by the nickname Dentatus. Pliny stated in the case of females, the presence of teeth at birth did not bode well for the future health. Others said to have been born with natal teeth include Zoroaster, Hannibal, and King Richard III of England. France's Sun King, Louis XIV, was born with three teeth, causing "a considerable vexation to his wet nurse," and leading a Dutch savant, Hugo Grotius, to prophesize that Louis would be a great despoiler, which proved to be an accurate prediction. Richelieu, Mazarin, and Mirabeau, the esteemed orator, were other French said to be similarly endowed.

Shakespeare makes reference to the condition in *King Henry VI*," in Glouster's reminiscence:

> *For I have often heard my mother say*
> *I came into the world with my legs forward:*
> *Had I not reason, think ye, to make haste,*
> *And seek their ruin that usurp'd our right?*
> *The midwife wondered: and the women cried,*
> *O Jesus bless us, he is born with teeth!*
> —Part Third, Act V, Sc. 6

Shed-tooth rituals have taken a variety of forms, and often involved supplicating creatures known for their strong choppers to replace the lost tooth with a strong, permanent one.

In ancient Abyssinia, the child was instructed to throw the tooth to a howling hyena, and put in a request for strong teeth. In America, a Cherokee child ran around the house with the shed tooth, then threw it on the roof, saying four times, "Beaver put a new tooth in my jaw." Among the Chippewa, it fell on parents to do the honors, blackening the tooth with charcoal, throwing it to the west, and supplicating the child's grandmother to let another tooth grow. The practices merged in the Obijibwa, where the tooth was thrown to the east, with charcoal on it, and the parent ran around the house. The Teton Indians buried a child's tooth under the entrance to the lodge. People who walked over the tooth would then grow new teeth. Shuswap children would place a lost tooth in meat and feed it to a dog, saying, "Make my teeth strong." To develop strong teeth in Australia, mothers were taught to eat the teeth, after pounding them and placing in meat.

A form of vermin idolatry has also had a long association with shed teeth. With its sharp teeth, the mouse was a commanding figure from a dental prospective, and was often called upon to replace a lost tooth with a stronger one. (Mice were also regarded as channelers of sorts, able to communicate with departed ancestors on behalf of the living.) Thus, people threw primary teeth over their shoulders, out of windows, and out of the houses, all the while supplicating a mouse with variations of a theme expressed in one ritual as "Mousie, mousie, here you have a tooth, now give me another." The French custom called for throwing the lost tooth under the bed with a request for the mouse to eat the old tooth and bring the child a new one.

A subtle transition began to occur in the late nineteenth century. In a variation of the ritual in France, the mouse no longer replaced the tooth, but traded it for a small gift. French children waited for a nocturnal visit from *le petit souris,* the little mouse, when they wanted to cash in a lost tooth. The tooth was put in the child's shoe, and while the child slept, the mouse exchanged it for a coin. A barter system also developed wherein a sleeping youngster could trade a tooth for candy, not with a mouse but with a good fairy.

The mercantile aspect of the shed-tooth ritual achieved its florescence in the twentieth century with the appearance of the tooth fairy. Believed to be a totally American invention, the first known mention of the tooth fairy in print appears in an eponymous children's play of 1927. However, the tooth fairy ritual was apparently already in place by that time. As almost every youngster knows, the custom called for placing a shed baby tooth under a pillow, after which the tooth fairy exchanged it for a coin.

The short history of this noble sprite is documented at the privately owned Tooth Fairy Museum in Deerfield, Illinois. Curator Rosemary Wells, Ph.D., of the Northwestern University Dental School, has collected over 500 tooth fairy figurines and portraits along with a library of books about the ethereal elfette.

According to Dr. Wells, the tooth fairy is only known to exist in the United States and in countries with American enclaves. Most cultures of the world still invoke animals rather than imaginary creatures in their shed-tooth rituals. Yet no matter what her origin, we can now say definitively the tooth fairy is a real doll: In 1994, Mattel produced a tooth fairy Barbie.

Clearing the Air

TODAY ADVERTISEMENTS ISSUE imprecations against bad breath in all its variants. Our medicine cabinets and drugstore shelves bulge with mints, sprays, mouthwashes, gums, and drops to conquer these odors from the dawn's morning mouth to the midnight hour. Yet this oral odor fixation is long-standing. Bad breath has been offending people for millennia, and preoccupation with its amelioration is likewise a proud ancient tradition.

An Assyrian medical text offered advice on the subject, recommending careful cleansing of the teeth to avoid bad breath. Detailed instructions were offered on using the index finger, cloth, and salt to prevent the problem. Pliny, known for his dubious historical reporting, sounded surprisingly believable when he addressed this topic.

"A man's breath," he wrote, "becomes infected by the bad quality of the food, by the bad state of his teeth, and still more by old age. Experience teaches that against the bad odor of the breath it is useful to wash the mouth with pure wine before sleeping, and that to avoid aching of the teeth it is a good thing to rinse the mouth in the morning with several mouthfuls of fresh water."

The modern era of bad breath began in 1920. That was the year the manufacturer of Listerine, Warner Lambert, manufactured a scary-sounding condition to help market their product: halitosis. The term was reportedly exhumed from an old medical dictionary, and its scientific sound helped remove some of the "coarseness" out of a discussion of bad breath. The company also used an advertising campaign based on the public's infatuation with newspaper personal-interest stories and advice to the lovelorn columns. Each ad was a brief melodrama starring a temporary victim of halitosis and the social shame it caused. Readers could identify with and vicariously suffer the protagonist's loss of love, happiness, and success. And now they had the knowledge to assure a similar fate never befell them.

Though it has been with us all this time, today the perception of bad breath seems to be changing from social nuisance to health hazard. Dentists are gearing up to begin treating breath disorders. A growing number of breath-treatment centers and breath clinics promise prompt diagnosis and treatment using sophisticated instrumentation such as the Halimeter.

The good news about bad breath is that experts say many more people think they have it than actually do. Yet there is more than enough to go around, affecting an estimated 25 to 85 million Americans. Food, medicines, tobacco, and disease, all are capable of triggering bad breath. Most cases are temporary, such as that caused by consumption of garlic or raw onions. Their volatile oils are absorbed in the blood and exhaled through the lungs.

The majority of chronic cases of halitosis are ultimately created by fumes of volatile sulfur compounds (VSC), odorous gases like hydrogen sulfide (which smells like rotten eggs), fatty acids, ammonia, and methylmercaptan. These gases are by-products of digestive activity of anaerobic bacteria, such as fusobacterium and actinomyces. Though essential to digestion and common to all alimentary canals, they exist in greater numbers in those with bad breath. However, halitosis does not originate in the stomach, but in the mouth, where these bacteria reside. Studies at the University of Michigan have sniffed out the tongue as their primary home.

Eradicating the bacteria can be problematic for individuals with what dentists call "geographic tongue," whose irregular surface resembles the unruly contours of the Earth itself. Within the cracks and crevices, untold numbers of these bacteria, each a tiny halitosis factory, dwell.

The $1 billion worth of over-the-counter remedies Americans buy every year are of limited value in controlling bad breath. Antibacterial rinses, along with good, old-fashioned tongue scraping are recommended weapons. Chlorine dioxide is another germicide used for tongue-tied halitosis. Mouthwashes of the future may target specific bacteria, designed for an individual's particular oral chemistry.

For now, such is its stigma that halitosis can reportedly be fatal—at least among those who don't have it. In 20 percent of the imagined cases brought to professional attention, the individual's concern has reached the level of a social phobia, according to one expert, and some of them are at risk of suicide.

Frightful Facts

EVEN AS PAIN has been conquered, the caries routed, our oldest oral affliction remains: dental phobia. As in the days of the primitive tooth-drawer, many avoid encounters with oral-care providers completely. According to contemporary studies, 8 percent to 15 percent of the United States population is phobic about dental care. Of the remaining numbers, many exhibit or express some degree of dental anxiety, or fear of dentists.

How does this fear develop? The negative image of dentists as paragons of pain production, ceaselessly peddled by the media, doesn't help, but many cases are iatrogenic—that is, they result from treatment itself. One traumatic experience at the hands of a dentist can have lifelong consequences.

The fear may also result from feelings of loss of control or help-lessness at being laid out in supine position and having one's body entered. Unrealistic fears of the dangers of choking, gagging, and sharp instruments also figure in this phobia. Dentists' use of mask and gloves, common to current barrier techniques of office hygiene, can also pro-voke anxiety.

When phobics must seek oral care due to a dental emergency, their fear may be expressed by regression, sometimes to an infantile level, hysterical reactions, delusions, even physiologic disturbances such as fluctuations in immunity to infection, endocrine disturbances, and changes in salivary flow and chemistry consistent with clinical de-pression.

Treatment of phobic patients has traditionally involved "pharma-cologic modalities," that is, drugging patients into a stupor from which they are oblivious to what is being done to them. Now, however, behavioral-modification techniques are increasingly employed. Half-a-dozen dental phobia clinics across the United States, like the Dental Fear Treatment Network at the University of Kentucky in Lexington and the Dental Phobia Clinic at Mt. Sinai Medical Center in New York City, offer treatment for these patients' oral and mental problems.

Tools like the Corah Dental Anxiety Scale and the Mount Sinai Dental Fear Inventory help dentists gauge each individual's unique form of phobia and design customized plans for overcoming it. System-atic desensitization to the fear-producing stimuli and relaxation tech-niques are the primary methods of treatment. Success rates of 90 percent have been claimed by these programs.

Perhaps phobic patients can take some comfort in knowing they aren't the only ones frightened by their office visits. Treating anxious subjects is recognized as a common source of stress for most dentists, as well.

Mind Over Mouth

EFFORTS AT BEHAVIORAL modification and a more holistic approach to oral health care are indicative of dentists' growing appreciation for the psychological significance of the oral cavity. The stimulation of the mouth's soft tissues and subconscious feelings of pleasure and/or frustration and anxiety they can provoke are now recognized as having profound implications for dentistry.

As one text stated, "The mouth was the area of the body that very early in life was involved with feelings of pleasure and satisfaction during feeding or with frustration and anger if the feeding was late or difficult. The mouth is an area of the body that may be involved with sexual sensations. The mouth is used to show the expression of an emotion that a person is feeling. . . . Dental treatment and manipulation in the mouth may allow the patients to become aware of many of these feelings related to the mouth. For example, if as an infant the patient was frustrated and angry because of difficulty in feeding, these feelings may be "activated" during a dental visit and expressed as anger toward the dentist. Sexual feelings also may be activated by dental manipulations and, depending on the patient's feelings, a degree of satisfaction regarding sexual needs, affection, or anger may be misdirected to the dentist."

Or, as *Psychodynamics in Dental Practice* states, ". . . the mouth may be viewed as an area which fulfills conditions for experiencing both the inside and outside world, and is the only localized perceptual zone which includes in itself both the characteristics of interior and exterior perception. The mouth is simultaneously both an *interceptor* and *exterioceptor.* . . . Thus, the mouth may be viewed as the cradle of, and the basic model for, all external perception."

Yet how different is this well-considered view from the doctrine proclaimed by the decidedly less scholarly Holistic Dental Association: "The human organism is an integrated, bio-cybernetic entity and is incapable of being treated as separate components."

As we can see, dentistry has become much more complex than the term *oral care* previously implied. This awareness brings us closer to reaching an accommodation with this sometimes vexing cavity, to reconciling mankind's love-hate relationship with his teeth and his oral-care provider, and finally achieve a better understanding of the Manichaean nature of our mouths and ourselves.

Selected Bibliography

Ambler, Henry L., *Around the World Dentistry*, Cleveland, OH: Judson Printing Co., 1910.

Ambler, Henry L., *Facts, Fads and Fancies About the Teeth*, Cleveland, OH: Helman-Taylor Co., 1900.

Andreana, Sebastiano; Andreana, Giuseppe; Gonzalez, Yola; and Ciancio, Sebastian, "Thomas Berdmore, Dentist of His Majesty George III, and Dental Calculus," *Journal of the History of Dentistry*, Vol. 44, No. 3, Nov. 1996.

Berry, James H., "Questionable Care: What Can Be Done About Dental Quackery?", *Journal of the American Dental Association*, Vol. 115, Nov. 1987.

Boland, Frank K., *The First Anesthetic; the Story of Crawford Long*, Athens, GA: Univ. of Georgia Press, 1950.

Brain, Peter, *Galen on Bloodletting: A Study of the Origins, Development and Validity of His Opinions, with a Translation of the Three Works*, New York, Cambridge Univ. Press, 1986.

Bremner, M. D. K., *The Story of Dentistry from the Dawn of Civilization to the Present*, third ed., rev., Brooklyn: Dental Items of Interest Publishing Co., 1954.

Campbell, J. Menzies, *Dentistry Then and Now*, third ed. Glasgow, UK: Bell & Bain Ltd., 1981.

Carter, Bill; Butterworth, Bernard; Carter, Joseph G.; and Carter, John W., *Ethnodentistry and Dental Folklore*, Overland Park, KS: Folklore Books of Kansas City, 1987.

Carter, Joseph G., and Carter, Bill, *Folk Dentistry: A Cultural Evolution of Folk Remedies for Toothache*, Chapel Hill, NC: Author-Produced, 1990.

Carter, Joseph G., and Carter, Bill, *Herbal Dentistry: Herbal Dental Remedies from Ancient Time to the Present Day*, Chapel Hill, NC: Author-produced, 1990.

Cigrand, Bernard J., *The Rise, Fall and Revival of Dental Prosthesis*, Chicago, IL: Periodical Pub. Co., 1893.

Dobson, Jessie, *Barbers and Barber Surgeons of London*, Oxford, UK: Oxford University Press, 1979.

Dummett, Clifton O., and Dummett, Lois D., *Afro-Americans In Dentistry: Sequence and Consequence of Events,* Los Angeles: Clifton O. Dummett, 1978.

Eames, Gaspar, and Mohler, "The Mercury Enigma in Dentistry," *Journal of the American Dental Association,* Vol. 92, June 1976.

Fauchard, Pierre, *The Surgeon Dentist, or a Treatise on the Teeth,* second ed., 1746, translated by Lilian Lindsay, Pound Ridge, NY: Milford House 1969.

Foley, Gardner P., *Foley's Footnotes,* Wallingford, PA: Washington Square East Publishers, 1972.

Garfield, Sydney, *Teeth, Teeth, Teeth: A Treatise on Teeth and Related Parts of Man, Land and Water Animals from Earth's Beginning to the Future of Time,* New York: Simon and Schuster, 1969.

Geshwind, Max, "Strobelberger's De Dentium Podagra of 1630," *Journal of the History of Dentistry,* Vol. 44, No. 1, Mar. 1996.

Geshwind, Max "Wig-Maker, Barber, Bleeder and Tooth-Drawer," *Journal of the History of Dentistry,* Vol. 44, No. 3, Nov. 1996.

Glenner, Richard A.; Davis, Audrey; and Burns, Stanley, *The American Dentist: A Pictorial History with a Presentation of Early Dental Photography in America,* Missoula, MT: Pictorial Histories Publishing Co., 1990.

Glenner, Richard A., *The Dental Office: A Pictorial History,* Missoula, MT: Pictorial Histories Publishing Co., 1984.

Glenner, Richard A., "How It Evolved: Sit-Down Dentistry," *Journal of the History of Dentistry,* Vol. 44, No. 1, Mar. 1996.

Glenner, Richard A., "The Modern Reclining Dental Chair," *Journal of the History of Dentistry,* Vol. 44, No. 3, Nov. 1996.

Goldman, Harriet; Hartman, Kenton; and Messite, Jacqueline, *Occupational Hazards in Dentistry,* Chicago: Year Book Medical Publishers, 1984.

Guerini, Vincinzo, *A History of Dentistry from the Most Ancient Times Until the End of the Eighteenth Century,* Philadelphia: Lea & Febiger, 1909.

Hillam, Christine, "Robert Wooffendale, The Making of a Reputation," *Bulletin of the History of Dentistry,* Vol. 41, No. 1, Mar. 1993.

Hillam, Christine, Ed., the Lindsay Society for the History of Dentistry, *The Roots of Dentistry,* London: British Dental Association, 1990.

Hoffmann-Axthelm, Walter, *History of Dentistry,* Chicago: Quintessence Publishing Co., 1981.

Holbrook, Stewart H., *The Golden Age of Quackery,* New York: Macmillan, 1959.

Hubbell, Sue, "Let Us Now Praise the Romantic, Artful, Versatile Toothpick," *Smithsonian,* Vol. 27, No. 10, Jan. 1997.

Jameson, Eric, *The Natural History of Quackery,* London: M. Joseph, 1961.

Kanner, Leo, *Folklore of the Teeth,* New York: Macmillan, 1928.

Kells, Charles Edmund, *Three Score Years and Nine*, New Orleans: Edmund Kells, 1926.

Kiple, Kenneth F. (ed.), Graham, Rachael R. (exec. ed), Frey, David (assoc. ed.) et al., *The Cambridge World History of Human Disease*, Cambridge, UK: Cambridge University Press, 1993.

Koch, Charles R. E., *History of Dental Surgery*, Fort Wayne, IN: National Art Publishing Co., 1910.

Krochak, Michael, "An Overview of the Treatment of Anxious and Phobic Dental Patients," *Compendium of Continuing Education of Dentistry*, Vol. XIV, No. 5, May 1993.

Lufkin, Arthur, *A History of Dentistry*, second ed., Philadelphia: Lea & Febiger, 1948.

Maier, Franz J., *Fluoridation*, Cleveland: CRC Press, 1972.

McCluggage, Robert W., *A History of the American Dental Association; a Century of Health Service*, Chicago: American Dental Association, 1959.

Miller, Ronald D., *Anesthesia*, New York: Churchill Livingstone, 1994.

Monica, Woodrow S., *Outline of Dental History*, Hackensack, NJ: Farleigh Dickinson University Dental School, 1972.

Nevius, Laird W., *The Discovery of Anaesthesia: By Whom Was It Made? A Brief Statement of Facts*, New York: G. W. Nevius, 1894.

Ogg, Frederic A., *Daniel Webster*, Philadelphia: G. W. Jacobs & Co., 1914.

Ottolengni, Rodrigues, *Table Talks on Dentistry*, New York: Dental Items of Interest Publishing Co., 1935.

Park, Edwards, "The Object at Hand," *Smithsonian*, Vol. 27. No. 12, Mar. 1997.

Porter, Roy, *Health for Sale: Quackery in England 1660–1850*, Manchester, UK: University Press; New York: St. Martin's Press, 1989.

Prinz, Hermann, *Dental Chronology*, Philadelphia: Lea & Febiger, 1945.

Pronych, Peter M., and Christen, Arden C., "Painless Parker: A Dental Renegade's Fight to Make Advertising Ethical," Baltimore, MD: Distributed for the American Academy of the History of Dentistry, 1995.

Proskauer, Curt, and Witt, Fritz H., *Pictorial History of Dentistry*, Koln, Germany: M Du Mont Schaubert, 1962.

Protell, Martin R.; Krasner, Jack D.; and Fabrikant, Benjamin, *Psychodynamics in Dental Practice*, Springfield, IL: Charles C. Thomas, 1975.

Ring, Malvin E., *Dentistry: An Illustrated History*, New York: Harry S. Abrams; St. Louis, MO: C. V. Mosby Co., 1985.

Ring, Malvin E., "Do-it-Yourself Dentistry," *Bulletin of the History of Dentistry*, Vol. 41, No. 1, Mar. 1993.

Ring, Malvin E., "Is Teething a Disease? Mixed Feelings of 130 Years Ago," *Bulletin of the History of Dentistry*, Vol. 42, No. 1, Mar. 1994.

Ring, Malvin E., "The Rubber Denture Murder Case, the True Story of Vulcanite Litigations," *Journal of the History of Dentistry*, Vol. 32, No. 1, Apr. 1984.

Robinson, J. Ben, *Foundations of Professional Dentistry*, Baltimore: Waverly Press, 1940.

Rubin, J. G., *Dental Phobia and Anxiety*, Philadelphia: W. B. Saunders, 1988.

Rubin, J. G.; Slovin, Mark; and Krochak, Michael, "The Psychodynamics of Dental Anxiety and Dental Phobia," *Dental Clinics of North America*, Vol. 28, No. 4, Oct. 1988.

Sava, George, *The Conquest of Pain: The Story of Anaesthesia*, London: MacDonald, 1946.

Smith, Truman, and Ellsworth, Pickeny W., *An Inquiry into the Origin of Modern Anaesthesia*, Hartford, CT: Brown and Gross, 1867.

Taylor, James A., *History of Dentistry; a Practical Treatise for the Use of Dental Students and Practitioners*, Philadelphia and New York: Lea & Febiger, 1922.

Thompson, Charles J. S., *The Quacks of Old London*, New York and London: Brentano's, 1928.

Weinberger, Bernhard W., *An Introduction to the History of Dentistry, with Medical and Dental Chronology and Bibliographic Data*, St. Louis: C. V. Mosby Co., 1948.

Wiley, P.; Glenner, Richard A.; and Scott, Douglas D., "Oral Health of Seventh Cavalry Troopers: Dentitions from the Custer National Cemetery," *Journal of the History of Dentistry*, Vol. 44, No. 1, Mar. 1996.

Woodforde, John, *The Strange Story of False Teeth*, London: Routledge & K. Paul, 1968.

Young, James H., "American Health Quackery: Collected Essays," Princeton, NJ: Princeton University Press, 1992.

Young, James H., "*The Long Struggle Against Quackery in Dentistry*," *Journal of the History of Dentistry*, Vol. 33, No. 3, Oct. 1985.

Young, James H., *The Medical Messiahs; A Social History of Health Quackery in Twentieth Century America*, Princeton, NJ: Princeton University Press, 1967.

Index